My Resilient Win

How a 10-Year-Old Boy Defeated Inflammatory Bowel Disease Without Prescription Drugs or Surgery

Bradley Collier

Bradley Collier presents:

My Resilient Win: How a 10-Year-Old Boy Defeated Inflammatory Bowel Disease Without Prescription Drugs or Surgery.

Copyright © 2024 by Bradley Collier. All rights reserved.

Except as allowed by the U.S. Copyright Act of 1976, no part of this book may be duplicated, saved in a retrieval system, communicated, or distributed in any way without the publisher's express written consent.

The publisher is not responsible for websites, or their content not owned by the publisher.

Library of Congress Cataloging-in-Production Data
    Collier, Bradley.
My Resilient Win: How a 10-year-old boy defeated inflammatory bowel disease without prescription drugs or surgery / Bradley Collier.
First Edition.
    p. cm.
ISBN 979-8-218-46286-4 (paperback)
ISBN 979-8-332-40659-1 (hardcover)

1. Inflammatory Bowel Disease (IBD). 2. Ulcerative Colitis. 3. Health. 4. The Specific Carbohydrate Diet. 5. Winning Despite Adversity – Nonfiction. 6. Self-Help. 7. Motivational & Inspirational.   I. Title.

2024913025

10 9 8 7 6 5 4 3 2 1

Bradley Collier, West Palm Beach, Florida

For Nana

Good Health

Contents

Author's Note 1
Acknowledgements 3
1. A Punch in The Gut.. 11
2. Upper Endoscopy and Colonoscopy 21
3. Ulcerative Colitis.. 29
4. Autoimmune Diseases 39
5. Allergies 43
6. The Specific Carbohydrate Diet 47
7. Meal Planning 63
8. Butternut Squash Fries 69
9. Dining Out.. 75
10. Managing Food Cravings 81
11. Strategies for Staying Symptom Free..................... 89
12. The Importance of Exercise 93
13. My Special Hydration Formula: Bradleyaid 101
14. Alternative Treatments 105
15. I Defeated Ulcerative Colitis 107
My Resilient Win 116
A Preview of My Next Book 121
References 126
About the Author 130

Author's Note

In my opinion, too many people suffer from poor health. Genetics can play a part, but for many, poor health isn't simply because of genetic factors. Wealth and environmental factors can impact one's health. Also, the combination of poor eating habits and a lack of physical activity can lead to poor health. Psychological factors can also contribute to poor health. A tragedy is many negative health circumstances can be prevented.

    I wrote *My Resilient Win* to help and inspire people to transition to better health. I have inflammatory bowel disease (IBD), and I've defeated it through lifestyle changes. This, despite there being no known cure for inflammatory bowel disease! IBD is one of many types of autoimmune diseases which have reached epidemic levels.[1]

---

[1] Olivia Casey and Frederick W. Miller, "Autoimmunity Has Reached Epidemic Levels. We Need Urgent Action to Address it." Scientific American, A Division of Springer Nature America, Inc., December 1, 2023. https://www.scientificamerican.com/article/autoimmunity-has-reached-epidemic-levels-we-need-urgent-action-to-address-it/

MY RESILIENT WIN

Inflammatory bowel disease (IBD) is an "umbrella term for two conditions that cause chronic inflammation in the digestive system: ulcerative colitis and Crohn's disease."[1] "Both ulcerative colitis and Crohn's disease usually are characterized by diarrhea, rectal bleeding, abdominal pain, fatigue and weight loss."[2]

Inflammatory bowel disease and other autoimmune diseases are a challenge for millions of people. I hope *My Resilient Win* helps people overcome challenges on their journey toward achieving optimal health and success in life.

-Bradley Collier

---

[1] "Inflammatory Bowel Disease," Yale Medicine, accessed online July 26, 2024, https://www.yalemedicine.org/conditions/inflammatory-bowel-disease

[2] Mayo Clinic Staff, "Inflammatory bowel disease (IBD)," Mayo Clinic, September 3, 2022, https://www.mayoclinic.org/diseases-conditions/inflammatory-bowel-disease/symptoms-causes/syc-20353315

Acknowledgements

I thank God, my parents, grandparents, doctors, and friends. I thank those who shared their stories about inflammatory bowel disease, and those who shared solutions for improving one's health. This has helped me become healthy. I thank Master Han of U.S. Pro Taekwondo in Jupiter, Florida. I started training in Taekwondo at 5 years old. The lessons learned in Taekwondo help me deal with the ups and downs of life. If I get knocked down, I will get up and fight.

  I give a big thanks to Jack and Jill of America, Inc., and the Palm Beach Chapter for nurturing future leaders through their many great programs and conferences. They gave me a chance to meet many amazing professionals, government leaders, and even astronauts. I am thankful for the great friendships I've made and the opportunities to provide service to my community. Jack and Jill of America, Inc., has enhanced my life in countless ways. For instance, the national cultural exchange trip to Greece in 2023 was a life changing experience.

MY RESILIENT WIN

    I thank my basketball trainers, Coach Ashton Khan, who my mom found during the global pandemic. Thanks for the life lessons you taught me and making me a better human being, student, and basketball player. If I can do two things with a basketball, it's handle the ball and make three pointers. The strength and conditioning routine you created for me helped take me to a new level.

    I thank Coaches Brian Macon, Marvens Calixte and the team at Handlelife. Working with trainers who train many NBA players allowed me to understand that basketball is more than a game. Basketball helped teach me resilience! It's a game full of mistakes. You will face adversity in basketball and life. One must be resilient to overcome adversity. It was really cool meeting NBA All-Star Scottie Barnes at your camp. It was also awesome when the NBA Morris twins (Marcus and Markeiff) stopped by your growth program and told me to keep working. Your impact in my life goes far beyond the basketball court.

    Thanks to Coach Lance Thomas. Those early basketball lessons you gave me and C.J. at the park helped foster my love of the game. Thanks to Coach Justin Murray for perfecting my shooting form. Thanks to Coach Lorenzo Hands. I can't express how grateful I am for the things you gave me from Michael Jordan's basketball camp. And thanks to Coach Nate Vera and the Perseverance Basketball family. Playing for Coach Clayton Williams was awesome, and Coach Brandon Mycal fixed my defensive footwork, making me a much better defender.

    I thank my teachers, the administration, and fellow students at Suncoast Community High School in Riviera Beach, Florida. Suncoast is one of the best high schools in

Acknowledgements

the U.S.[1] The curriculum is so difficult, I had to learn time management and how to study intensely. Being around elite students helps motivate me to strive for academic excellence. Having taken many AP classes, I know I'm ready to do well academically in college.

I want to give a huge thanks to Ms. Olive Bryan, Ms. Brittany Rigdon, and the whole team at Excelsior College Planning. Your tutoring made me a better student, and I wouldn't have achieved the AP Scholar with Distinction Award without your amazing coaching. Thank you so much!

I thank Chef Shannon Atkins, who makes my family's life much easier. Chef Shannon's phenomenal meals are a blessing.

I thank Celebrity Sports Academy for their great camps, which taught me many things and gave me priceless, lifelong memories. I still can't believe I got to meet Dwyane Wade and Jimmy Butler.

I also thank Elaine Gottschall for writing *Breaking the Vicious Cycle: Intestinal Health Through Diet*, which introduced me to the specific carbohydrate diet.

I didn't know how hard it is to write a book until I started writing *My Resilient Win*. My parents reminded me of how many people I would help, and that inspired me to fight to complete *My Resilient Win*. Without resilience and a positive mental attitude, there is no way I could have defeated inflammatory bowel disease.

---

[1] "2024 Best U.S. High Schools," U.S. News & World Report, accessed online April 10, 2024, https://www.usnews.com/education/best-high-schools/florida/districts/the-school-district-of-palm-beach-county/suncoast-community-high-school-5380

My Resilient Win

*Resilient through the trauma
resilience and time
if I am resilient
all will be fine*

                    -Bradley Collier

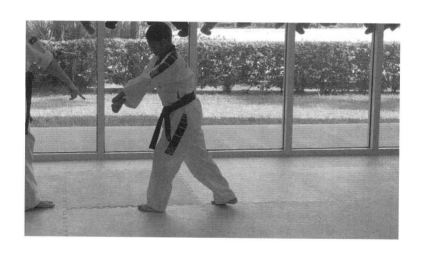

Chapter 1
A Punch in The Gut

Hello, my name is Bradley Collier. At ten years old, after going through a series of tests and having two medical procedures (a colonoscopy and upper endoscopy), I received a life changing diagnosis: I have ulcerative colitis! At the time I wrote this book, this autoimmune disease has no known cure, and I'll possibly have it for the rest of my life. However, I healed myself. I have no symptoms of the disease and don't take any medication for ulcerative colitis. I did this through no feat of magic, though it did take an extreme level of discipline, as I'll explain.

Like me, you probably see lots of television commercials for ulcerative colitis medication. I find these commercials quite alarming. What I also find alarming is some of the side effects of many of these medications.

MY RESILIENT WIN

"According to the Centers for Disease Control and Prevention (CDC), an estimated 3.1 million people in the United States have some form of IBD, and the number is steadily rising."[1]

I was once very sick with ulcerative colitis and felt miserable. But now I'm healthy and happy. I'm a good student, good athlete, and have lots of energy. I'm six foot three inches tall with an athletic build and can dunk a basketball. I run track and am a second-degree international black belt in Taekwondo. My future looks bright.

Over several years, I've taken tests for even the smallest trace of inflammatory bowel disease, and all tests have come back negative. I've healed from within due to a lifestyle change.

How it all started

As a fourth grader, I was having a great day. School was fun and now I could focus on having more fun at home. Like most days, I was playing with my toys without a care in the world, other than having more fun.

Suddenly, my stomach started to hurt really bad. I felt like I had to poop, so I interrupted my playtime and walked to the nearest bathroom. I took a poop without any straining, but my stomach felt like I'd done a whole lot of sit-ups. My stomach burned like I'd torn some muscles. When I wiped my bottom, I discovered blood on the toilet

---

[1] "Can modern lifestyle affect chances of inflammatory bowel disease?" Medical News Today, Last medically reviewed on March 13, 2024. https://www.medicalnewstoday.com/articles/320283

paper. Then I looked at my poop and it was covered with blood, a bright red, scary-looking blood. There was something else strange looking about my poop. Something was mixed throughout my poop, and I didn't know what it was. This is awful, I thought. I was creeped out and scared, like horror movie scared.

I yelled "daddy, daddy! There's blood in my poop!"

My dad yelled, "I'll be right there," and in a moment my dad said, "open the door."

I stood out of the way so there was enough room to open the door without hitting me. My dad looked at my poop and said "wow," and then he paused and just stared. By this time, some of the water in the toilet was turning bloody.

My dad had his phone in his pocket, so he pulled it out and took a picture.

"Finish wiping yourself, but do it very softly," he said. "I don't know if you have a cut in your butt or not."

I wiped myself gently and my butt didn't hurt. I continued to wipe myself gently, until there was no poop or blood on the toilet paper. This isn't anything I'd experienced before. I guess it's natural I was frightened.

"What's that stuff in my poop?" I asked.

"It looks like mucus," my dad replied, "but I'll have to ask your mother. Don't worry, everything will be okay."

My dad flushed the toilet and told me to wash my hands. He then went to another bathroom and washed his hands. He told me he was going to send a text message to my mother about this.

I watched daddy as he sent a text message to my mom. I don't know exactly what he told her, or if he sent her a picture of my poop, but I was impatient and wanted to know how she replied. My mom is a doctor and she's smart. She had to know what's going on, I thought.

"What'd she say? What'd she say, daddy?" I asked, with my anxiety building.

My father said, "She's busy seeing patients; she'll answer me when she gets a chance."

A little later daddy explained mommy will call my doctor. We must monitor the situation and next time I poop, don't flush the toilet, and call him or mommy. Both want to see my poop, but at minimum, one of them must see it if the other isn't home.

My mom spoke with my pediatrician and scheduled an appointment. We were able to see him the next day. He's a great doctor in my opinion. My mom seemed nervous as we headed to my appointment, but my dad tried to calm her down.

My doctor was always in a pleasant mood. He examined me and asked me several questions. He said a possible cause for my bloody poop is a parasite. More specifically, an amoeba can cause a parasitic infection that can cause bloody poop.

My doctor ordered a test to see if there was an amoeba in my body. It took a few days for us to get the test results. In the meantime, like a ritual, every time I pooped, my mom or dad (or both) would look at it. After seeing my poop for a few days, there was no change. My poop was still bloody with mucus in it.

The test to see if I had an amoeba in my body came back negative, so this wasn't the cause of my bloody poop. Then my doctor referred me to a pediatric gastroenterologist. Now I was really getting scared.

Gastroenterology is "the branch of medicine that deals with the diagnosis and treatment of diseases and disorders of the digestive system." [1]

I could tell my mother was quite nervous. However, my father didn't seem nervous at all. Maybe my mom was nervous because she's a doctor, and maybe my dad wasn't nervous because he had no idea how severe my condition could be. Maybe it's because he's a man. I don't know, but he was cool as ice.

---

[1] "Gastroenterology," The Free Dictionary by Farlex, accessed online February 7, 2024 https://www.thefreedictionary.com/gastroenterology

MY RESILIENT WIN

When we arrived for my appointment with the gastroenterologist, before we got to see him, a medical assistant measured my height, weight, and took my blood pressure. Then we met the doctor, and he asked lots of questions. He also checked my heart rate, looked in my mouth, ears, and felt my tummy.

The doctor ordered multiple tests to try to find out why I was experiencing the symptoms I'd been having. He told me and my parents I might need a procedure called a colonoscopy, depending on the results of the tests. The doctor explained I had to go to a blood lab and have blood drawn. I also had to use a kit to collect a sample of my poop so it could be analyzed by a lab.

The Blood Lab

My mother scheduled an appointment with a blood lab, and it took a few days before I could get an appointment. My mom explained to me that I was going to have to have a needle stuck into my arm for a blood sample to be collected. I knew it was going to hurt.

On the morning of my appointment, I was really scared. I felt sick to my stomach, and I couldn't stop thinking about how much getting a needle stuck into me was going to hurt. I hate needles! My mom kept telling me it was going to be okay, but I was still nervous.

When we got to the lab, the smell of disinfectant hit me, and I got more scared. My mom held my hand, reassuring me that everything would be okay. She said we were there to make sure I was healthy, which made me feel a little better.

At the blood lab, a lab technician (a phlebotomy technician) greeted us and took us to a room where I could sit down. "Phlebotomy technicians collect blood from patients and prepare the samples for testing." [1]

The lab technician explained what she was going to do, but that didn't ease my mind. I was still scared, and for a good reason. I knew it was going to hurt when I got stuck with a needle.

My mom tried to keep me distracted by talking to me while the technician got everything ready. I tried to focus on how happy I'd be when we left the blood lab, and this helped me calm down.

When it was time to get poked with the needle, the lab technician took a big rubber band and tied it tightly around my arm. Then she used an alcohol swab to clean the area where she was going to stick the needle. I felt a painful pinch when she stuck the needle in my arm, but it wasn't as bad as I thought it would be. Then she took the rubber band off my arm. As the lab technician collected the blood samples, I tried to stay calm.

Finally, the lab technician took the needle out, and put a bandage on my arm. It was all over. What a relief! My mom told me I was brave, and I must be proud of myself.

I was very proud of myself!

---

[1] "Phlebotomy Technician," Mayo Clinic College of Medicine and Science, Mayo Foundation for Medical Education and Research., accessed online March 9, 2024, https://college.mayo.edu/academics/explore-health-care-careers/careers-a-z/phlebotomy-technician/

MY RESILIENT WIN

Leaving the lab, I felt like I had done something big, especially for a ten-year-old. Even though I was still a little scared, I knew I had faced my fears with mom by my side. And with the test results, I hoped we would find out what was wrong and how to make me feel better soon. Later that day when I saw my dad, he said, "Good job!"

The Poop Sample

My mother helped me get the poop sample. First, my mom placed a container that was supposed to collect my poop on the toilet in my bathroom. It was placed under the toilet's seat, but above the toilet bowl (the toilet seat held the container in place over toilet bowl). The container was tall enough to collect my poop, but not so tall that the bottom of it touched the water in the toilet.

When I had to poop, I let my mother know, and she stood outside of the door until I had pooped in the container. It was really embarrassing to have to poop in a container. When I was done pooping, I called my mother, and she entered the bathroom. She had to use a tool that looked like a small popsicle stick to pick up pieces of poop and put them in two separate containers. After this, she screwed a lid on top of the containers and placed them in a small plastic bag. The rest of the poop got flushed down the toilet and we threw away the container attached to the toilet seat. After this, my mom took the poop samples to a clinical lab so they could be tested.

After the lab checked out my poop samples, it turns out I had a ton of inflammation going on, but my gastroenterologist still didn't know why. We had to go back and see my gastro doc again so he could explain the test results and figure out why I was sick.

So, my gastro doc broke down the test results for us, and I didn't understand what he was talking about. Then he suggests I should get an upper endoscopy and a colonoscopy done. What? My gastro doc is a top expert on my symptoms and thinks these procedures will probably figure out what's causing all my weird symptoms.

Chapter 2

Upper Endoscopy and Colonoscopy

"What's a colonoscopy?" I asked the doctor.

He told me he was going to look inside my body with a small scope to see why I was sick. He said I'd be asleep when he did the procedure.

"Will it hurt?" I asked.

"No," the doctor replied.

He explained I'd have some numbing cream put on my hand, so an IV doesn't hurt when they put it in, and an anesthesiologist would put me to sleep. When I wake up, my gastro doc would be all done with the procedure. I had no idea what an IV is, but now I was overwhelmed so I didn't ask. I also didn't know what an anesthesiologist is, but at this point, I just wanted to go home.

Colonoscopies are rare for kids, but sometimes, when they can't figure out why you're sick, they'll suggest one. And yep, that's exactly what happened to me, since all the other tests didn't show why I was sick.

On the ride back home, my mom tried to explain things to me in more detail. She told me I'd also need to get an upper endoscopy done. That's where they slide this bendy tube with a camera on it down your throat to peek at your esophagus, stomach, and the start of your small intestine. They look for stuff like inflammation, ulcers, or tumors. Being 10, I was like, "Nope, don't want to know anymore," and barely got what she was talking about.

So, in a colonoscopy, they stick this tube-like thing called a colonoscope up your butt and into your colon. This lets the gastro doc check out the inside walls of your colon to see if there's any weird stuff like ulcers, growths, swelling, or even signs that could mean colorectal cancer.

As a vibrant and curious kid, I was concerned about my health. I hoped we would get all the info we needed so I could get better. I was scared after learning I was going to have a colonoscopy.

My mom explained that I was taking a day off from school to have the procedures. This is great, I thought. No school!

"Will it hurt?" I asked. I wanted to see if she said anything different from my gastro doc.

"No," my mother said. "They'll give you some medicine to put you to sleep. You won't feel a thing. Me and daddy will be there when you go to sleep, and we'll be there when you wake up."

Preparing for the colonoscopy

Man, this really sucked! The day before my colonoscopy was horrible. I had to drink a bunch of liquid prescribed by my gastro doc and do this thing called an enema. Basically, my mom had to help me squirt some liquid up my butt using a tube. Dang, this was messed up! The whole point was to clean out my colon, make me poop, and make the poop softer. Not exactly how I planned to spend my day, but yeah, that happened.

Don't complain and keep a positive mental attitude!

I didn't complain to my parents. My dad often says, "complaining only makes things worse." My dad had 14 surgeries (6 were emergencies) and he didn't complain once. He was still recovering from his most recent emergency, where he easily could have died. One day his intestine ruptured but he didn't feel any pain. He had some black marks on his skin that stung a little bit, and he showed mommy. Mommy made him go to the emergency room immediately while I was eating dinner. The real crazy thing is, he had just had another emergency surgery a month before this.

Daddy was in the hospital for 8 days. They fixed the hole in his intestine and took out his entire abdominal wall. A skillful surgeon replaced his abdominal wall with a collagen graft. That is, his new abdominal wall is made of pig skin. When he finally came home, he had a 9-inch slice on his stomach and was hooked to a big machine he had to carry around called a wound vac, which helped him heal. A nurse had to come to our house to change his bandages for

6 weeks. Even though he was in intense pain for a long time, he didn't complain. What daddy explained to me is you have to count your blessings and thank God you wake up each day. He told me it was better to be in pain than be dead. It takes about a year to fully recover from what daddy went through, but I don't think he ever fully recovered.

The Upper Endoscopy and Colonoscopy

The morning of my procedures, I couldn't eat or drink anything, but the good thing is, my procedures were early in the morning. This would give me more time to play later and enjoy a day off from school, I thought.

I could tell my mother was nervous, but my father wasn't nervous at all. My dad looked like he always does, ready to yell if he thought I did anything wrong, but otherwise, he was relaxed.

We arrived at the hospital well in advance of my procedures and I was very nervous. Me and my parents were taken to a waiting area, where I had to undress and put on a robe. Then I sat on a bed that had wheels. My mother told me that someone would roll me in the bed to the room where the doctor would meet us.

A nurse entered the room and told us she needed to set up an IV. The nurse grabbed my arm and was about to stick a needle into my wrist, but my father stopped her and asked, "Aren't you going to numb his hand first?"

The nurse replied, "I need to keep things on schedule."

As she prepared to stick a needle into my wrist. My father said, "I don't care about your schedule! He needs numbing cream before you stick that needle in him!"

Upper Endoscopy and Colonoscopy

I was confused. My doctor said they'd numb my hand. Also, I had a facetime call with my good friend C.J. and told him about my procedures. He told me they'd put numbing cream on me so the needle wouldn't hurt. It was clear to me the nurse didn't care how much pain I'd have to feel.

The nurse looked furious, but my father looked even more mad. The nurse walked off with a disgusted look on her face, and in a few minutes, she returned. She put some numbing cream on my wrist and said, "This will take a few minutes to numb your hand. I'll be back in a little while to set up the IV."

In about 15 minutes, the nurse returned and checked to confirm if my hand was numb enough to insert an IV without too much pain. My hand was quite numb, so the nurse inserted an IV, and thanks to the numbing cream, I didn't feel any pain. I'm glad my father insisted on numbing cream. He knows how much an IV can hurt.

My gastroenterologist stopped by to see how I was doing. He told me I won't feel a thing and both procedures combined should take about an hour. He said I should relax, and an anesthesiologist would be there soon to help me go to sleep.

A little while later an anesthesiologist spoke with me and my parents, then gave me a sedative as I got ready for my medical procedures. I was in a good mood now as I was very relaxed. Soon, medical staff started to roll my bed down a hallway as my parents walked beside the bed. The last thing I saw was my gastroenterologist smiling before I fell asleep.

The next thing I knew, I was waking up. It seemed as if I had just fallen to sleep a few moments earlier. Wow, that was quick, I thought. I felt quite drowsy as I laid in a recovery area. I was surrounded by nurses and my relieved parents.

My parents told me I did a good job, they love me and are proud of me, then they hugged and kissed me.

Having medical procedures can be hard, especially if the patient is young. But my parents' support made the situation less stressful, particularly when my father stepped in to stop the nasty nurse from hurting me with an IV.

During the upper endoscopy and colonoscopy my gastroenterologist took biopsies of my esophagus, stomach, and colon. I'm glad he didn't try to do this while I was awake, or I'd have freaked out. A biopsy is when they take a bit of tissue and send it to a doctor called a pathologist, who checks it out and figures out what's going on.

Ulcerative Colitis Diagnosis

My gastroenterologist told my parents the results of my procedures while I was asleep. He found inflammation in my lower intestine and verified that I have ulcerative colitis (which the biopsies also confirmed later). The doctor advised my parents that with the right attention and medicines, I should heal quickly and get back to my regular life. He had many patients who did well with the right medication.

Upper Endoscopy and Colonoscopy

My parents seemed happy when I woke up and saw them, but I could tell my mother was worried. Since my mother is a doctor, she knew that ulcerative colitis is a lifelong condition and those with it have a very high risk of colon cancer. Many times, people must take medication for ulcerative colitis, and the meds stop working for them. Then patients are on a rollercoaster, moving from one medication to another throughout their life.

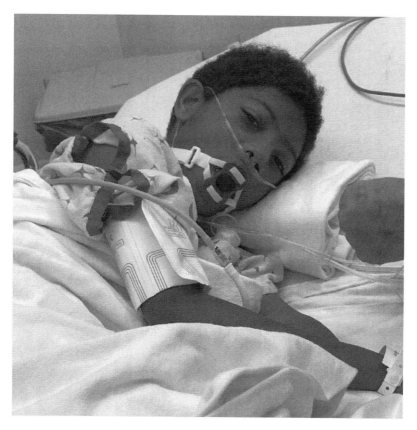

After I woke up following my procedures

MY RESILIENT WIN

I can't stress enough how important my endoscopy and colonoscopy were. Like, when you're dealing with stomach issues as a kid, it can really mess with your health. To dodge bigger problems down the line and keep growing strong, catching this stuff early and getting on top of treatment is super important.

You got to realize how hard this kind of medical stuff can hit you emotionally, especially as a kid. You might get over it physically, but it sticks with you and can be pretty rough. Making sure kids going through these procedures get all the emotional support and counseling they need is key. It makes getting back to normal life a lot smoother.

My gastroenterologist checked on me to see if I was okay before I could go home. He told me I'd get better soon. My parents waited until we were in the car to explain my diagnosis. I had a hard time understanding what was wrong with me but was happy to be done with my procedures. I remember going to eat at Wendy's on our way home. I was so happy to eat a cheeseburger and fries. We didn't know at this point how bad these could be for people with ulcerative colitis.

Chapter 3
Ulcerative Colitis

"Ulcerative colitis is an inflammatory bowel disease in which the inner lining of the large intestine and rectum become inflamed. Ulcerative colitis is characterized by diarrhea, abdominal pain and blood in the stool. The disease may vary in how much of the colon is affected and in severity as well."[1] "Ulcerative colitis and Crohn's disease are the two main forms of inflammatory bowel diseases."[2]

---

[1] "Ulcerative Colitis," The Johns Hopkins University, The Johns Hopkins Hospital, and Johns Hopkins Health System, accessed online June 3, 2024, https://www.hopkinsmedicine.org/health/conditions-and-diseases/ulcerative-colitis

[2] "Ulcerative Colitis vs Crohn's Disease," UCLA Health, accessed online June 3, 2024, https://www.uclahealth.org/medical-services/gastro/ibd/patient-resources/ulcerative-colitis-vs-crohns-disease

Since ulcerative colitis, or UC, is an autoimmune condition, your body is essentially attacking itself.

"Symptoms may include:

- Bloody diarrhea, often the main symptom of ulcerative colitis
- Frequent bowel movements
- Abdominal or rectal pain
- Fever
- Weight loss
- Joint pain
- Skin rashes
- Occasionally, constipation and rectal spasms"[1]

"The cause of ulcerative colitis is unknown. People with this condition have problems with their immune system. However, it is not clear if immune problems cause this illness. Stress and certain foods can trigger symptoms, but they do not cause ulcerative colitis." [2]

---

[1] "Ulcerative Colitis," The Johns Hopkins University, The Johns Hopkins Hospital, and Johns Hopkins Health System, accessed June 3, 2024, https://www.hopkinsmedicine.org/health/conditions-and-diseases/ulcerative-colitis

[2] "Ulcerative Colitis," Michael M. Phillips, MD, David Zieve, MD, MHA, Brenda Conway, Editorial Director, and the A.D.A.M., Editorial team, Penn Medicine, Philadelphia, PA, Last Reviewed on 2/6/2022, accessed online April 9, 2024, https://www.pennmedicine.org/for-patients-and-visitors/patient-information/conditions-treated-a-to-z/ulcerative-colitis

For me, the pain of ulcerative colitis felt like someone was punching me in the stomach continuously. I felt constant pressure on my stomach. This made it hard for me to ever relax and hard for me to sleep.

The way UC hits you can be all over the place. Sometimes it's chill, and you're in remission, but then it can go nuts and you have flare-ups where you have symptoms again. In really bad situations, you could end up with scary stuff like toxic megacolon, holes in your colon, or even a higher chance of getting colon cancer.

To figure out if someone has UC, doctors gotta look at your health background, check you out physically, run some blood tests, analyze your poop, and use stuff like colonoscopies and biopsies to get a closer look at what's going on inside your body.

The goal of treating UC is to keep the inflammation in check, decrease the symptoms, and keep things stable without flare-ups. Usually, this involves a bunch of medications like steroids, biologics and other meds to calm down your immune system and reduce inflammation. If meds don't work or they're messing you up with side effects, sometimes surgery to take out the damaged parts of your colon is the next step.

Besides medication, changing your diet, figuring out how to deal with stress, and staying physically active are often suggested. Doctors really must keep a close watch on you to adjust your treatments and make sure nothing strange or bad starts happening with the disease.

Even though there is currently no known cure for UC, many people with the illness enjoy active, fulfilling lives because of effective management strategies.

Medication

My mother was really upset about my diagnosis, and I had more appointments with my gastroenterologist. I was prescribed the drug Canasa as part of my treatment.

Canasa is supposed to improve UC symptoms in a few days to a few weeks. It basically calms down the inflammation in your colon and rectum area, which means less abdominal pain and stopping bleeding from the butt.

Here's the tricky part about Canasa: You have to stick it in your butt!

I had to place the Canasa medicine in my butt once per day. It's shaped like a rocket ship. My father would carefully place a towel on a bed (over a plastic garbage bag), and I'd have to lay down sideways with my pants down. The plastic garbage bag would make sure nothing leaked on the bed. He would have placed the plastic bag over the towel or not use a towel at all, but it's not comfortable laying on plastic, and dad wanted me to be as comfortable as possible. He would put on plastic gloves, take the medicine out of its box and carefully push the Canasa in my butt.

Sometimes putting Canasa in my butt hurt, even though my dad was careful. The Canasa melts at body temperature, but sometimes it would melt so fast the medicine would immediately leak out of my bottom. And sometimes after the medicine had been put in my butt, there would be delay, and the medicine would leak out of my butt as I walked, sat or slept. I was embarrassed and would cry myself to sleep many nights.

After I started using Canasa, in the beginning, one major downside was getting diarrhea a lot. Plus, I began dropping weight and feeling nauseous a lot. But despite all that, eventually Canasa made me feel better than I was feeling before I began using the medicine, even though I was still having flare-ups where I'd have some symptoms of UC.

Besides the whole diarrhea thing, my stomach was still killing me, and man, the gas wouldn't stop. And not just any gas, my farts could clear a big room. There were times I almost didn't make it to the bathroom in time, always feeling like I needed to dash there. Luckily, my school had bathrooms close to every classroom. But yeah, there was this super embarrassing moment when I let one rip in class, and my teacher got super mad, while most of the kids in class were laughing.

My farts were really wet and sometimes when I farted, some liquid poop would leak out because I had diarrhea so often. It was nasty having sticky poop in my underwear, especially at school, because it stank. I tried to clean up as much as possible, but dang this was nasty. When this happened, I had to go home early.

Near the end of fourth grade, I had a huge flare-up where I had to go to the bathroom at school constantly. I pooped more than 20 times that day and my butt and stomach felt really sore. I had to leave school early and couldn't go back until the inflammation in my colon calmed down.

When I returned to school, I was often scared I'd fart really loud and everyone would laugh at me. I was so scared I'd fart, and poop would leak out and my underwear would stick to my butt like superglue. I couldn't focus in school because I constantly worried about pooping in my pants. Psychologically, this was very hard to deal with.

I was ashamed of myself.

My Mindset

I was in complete misery because ulcerative colitis is horrible. My family, teachers and classmates could tell I was losing weight. I was so skinny some kids made fun of me. But I wasn't just skinny, I felt weak. It didn't matter how much food I ate, I was still losing weight and felt sick most of the time.

My mom told the mothers of my closest friends for support. Having good friends helped me through the trauma of dealing with UC. I needed this support to endure.

I'm an athlete and it was very difficult to participate in Taekwondo or basketball. I got tired easily and needed far more rest breaks than other kids. Prior to getting sick, I was always full of energy and had more stamina than any other kid on my teams or in my Taekwondo class.

My father stayed and watched me closely at every practice I had. If he felt I needed a break, he would make me sit out and hydrate myself with Gatorade or water, even if he upset the coach by making me take a break. "Frequent diarrhea from UC can reduce your body's fluids to the point where you become dehydrated."[1]

---

[1] Stephanie Watson, medically reviewed by Mikhail Yakubov, MD, "Ulcerative Colitis and Dehydration," Healthline Media, April 16, 2021, https://www.healthline.com/health/ulcerative-colitis/ulcerative-colitis-and-dehydration-what-to-know

With symptoms of ulcerative colitis, it's important to stay well hydrated. "You can fix mild dehydration by drinking extra water. If you don't get enough to drink and diarrhea continues, dehydration can become serious enough to damage your kidneys. It could even be life threatening."[1]

One coach got really upset when my father walked onto the basketball court at practice while the coach was talking and handed me a bottle of water. When the coach got upset, my father just looked at him as if to dare him to say anything. My father had told the coach I was sick and needed extra hydration, but either the coach forgot, or didn't care. It was one thing if this was higher level basketball and I was healthy, but this was a recreation league. Either way, your health is more important than a basketball practice.

A few days later I had a test at school and spent most of the class time in the bathroom, constantly going from my desk to the bathroom. Each time I returned to my desk from the bathroom, it was only a few moments before I felt like I was going to poop in my pants and had to return to the bathroom.

I almost didn't finish the test. Luckily it didn't take the entire class time, or I wouldn't have finished. After this episode, my mother called my gastro doc and completed several forms that enabled me to get extra time to take exams in case I had to use the bathroom for an extended time. Because of this, I was going to be able to complete any test, despite my symptoms.

---

[1] Ibid.

MY RESILIENT WIN

In the summer, my parents paid for a basketball camp I wanted to attend. I was excited about the first day and my father drove me to camp. I was so weak I couldn't even make it through the initial warm up. I tried my best, but I was too weak. I had gotten plenty of rest and ate a good breakfast, but I was still too weak.

The coaches at the camp were concerned because I had attended the camp in previous years and trained with the coaches throughout the year, but I just couldn't handle the physical activity. I was doing my best to try to participate but my dad decided it was time for us to leave. He told me that if I feel better tomorrow, I can return to the camp. He tried to cheer me up, but I was distraught. However, I felt even worse the next day. I ended up missing the entire week of camp. This was extremely depressing.

I was devastated!

I couldn't complete athletic drills I normally did well. I was so tired. This was when I realized how serious this condition is. I felt I'd have to quit basketball and Taekwondo due to my illness. It's hard to explain, but I felt like I was going to die. I asked my dad, "Daddy, am I going to die?" Then I started crying.

Daddy told me, "Everyone dies at some point, but you're not going to die anytime soon. Everything will be okay."

Daddy explained that I need to keep a positive mental attitude, continue to eat well, get enough sleep, and in time I will feel better.

Having a positive mental attitude is important!

Chapter 4
Autoimmune Diseases

Our bodies are like a huge puzzle made of organs, tissue, and small cells. Consider our immune system as an amazing bodyguard meant to keep us safe from all the harmful viruses and bacteria out there. But sometimes it becomes a little confused and begins fighting our own body as if it's an enemy. When the immune system can't distinguish between a friend and enemy, autoimmune disease can result.

"Doctors don't know exactly what causes the immune system to misfire. Yet some people are more likely to get an autoimmune disease than others." [1]

---

[1] Stephanie Watson, medically reviewed by Avi Varma, MD, MPH, AAVHIVS, FAAFP, "Everything to Know About Autoimmune Diseases," Healthline, March 4, 2024, https://www.healthline.com/health/autoimmune-disorders

MY RESILIENT WIN

There are lots of autoimmune diseases and they have a wide range of symptoms. Multiple sclerosis, lupus, rheumatoid arthritis, type 1 diabetes, sarcoidosis, vitiligo, and psoriasis are a few examples of autoimmune diseases. People can suffer major physical and psychological effects from autoimmune diseases. Autoimmune diseases are often referred to as autoimmune disorders.

Autoimmune diseases are on the rise and are being diagnosed more often. But there are lots of challenges in diagnosing and treating autoimmune diseases. These include the need for improved diagnostic methods and tools, prevention techniques and stronger therapies with fewer side effects. A lot of work must be done to improve the quality of life for people with autoimmune diseases.

My Mom and her hearing loss

My mom had been sick about a year before my ulcerative colitis diagnosis, having suddenly lost the hearing in one of her ears. She got her hearing back after going to an ear, nose and throat doctor for a diagnosis and treatment. This type of doctor is often called an ENT. Her sudden hearing loss was startling.

Mom was at work seeing patients and noticed she couldn't hear anything out of one of her ears. She sent a text message to my dad to explain this, and he asked her if her ear was clogged, like what happens to some people when they take a flight on an airplane.

Her ear did feel clogged, and mom told dad she felt tired, like she was getting sick. When she got home from work, she went straight to bed. Typically, when mom got home, she would help me with my homework and spend time with me, but she let my dad know she wasn't feeling well and had to sleep, so dad helped me with my homework that night.

After two days of feeling exhausted, my mom felt like she was going deaf in her right ear as her hearing had not improved. When she told daddy this, he insisted she see a specialist at once, even if she had to cancel all her patients that day.

My mom called a nearby ENT doctor who was nice enough to add her to his busy schedule on the same day as her call. Had mom not seen an ENT doctor, her hearing loss might have been permanent. My mother knew someone else this happened to, but that person didn't get fast treatment and suffered permanent hearing loss.

Doctors don't know for sure why sudden hearing loss happens, but it's a serious emergency. Many doctors think it might be caused by autoimmune disease. The main problem with my mom's hearing was there was inflammation in her inner ear. To fix this, she got painful steroid injections directly through her eardrum. Her hearing got better after each shot. An audiologist kept track of her hearing during her recovery, and now she has perfect hearing again.

My mom thought deeply about how she lost her hearing to see if it held any clues on my ulcerative colitis diagnosis, especially since I'd always been healthy. Was it because of my diet? I enjoyed potato chips, French fries, and candy. I would eat a bunch of lollipops after school, but I didn't consume nearly as much junk food as many kids I know. My mom's hearing loss had occurred during a period of significant stress, leading her to believe that stress might have been a factor. However, neither she nor her ENT doctor knows the exact cause.

Since mommy's surprise health scare, she embarked on a self-care and stress reduction regimen. She often speaks on self-care to help others.

After my diagnosis with ulcerative colitis, mommy started doing research on autoimmune diseases. She was used to doing intense biomedical research as a medical student and resident, working with MD/PhDs from the U.S. Department of Health and Human Services, National Institutes of Health.

Chapter 5

Allergies

How and why did I get ulcerative colitis? We set out to solve the riddles around my health. Sometimes ulcerative colitis is genetic, but no one in my family had it. Ulcerative colitis is also linked to psoriasis, which I developed around the same time I was diagnosed with ulcerative colitis.

My mother was depressed about my ulcerative colitis diagnosis and looked for how my diet might impact my disease. As mom worked to have good health, she had been seeing a holistic doctor. Her holistic doctor was a board-certified family medicine doctor who also practiced holistic medicine. She was fully credentialed, and mom trusted her. So, mom decided to take me to see the doctor, who'd possibly be able to help me.

"Holistic medicine is a form of healing that considers the whole person – body, mind, spirit, and emotions – in the quest for optimal health and wellness." [1]

After a thorough examination, the holistic doctor had me take a food sensitivity blood test. **The results showed I had a sensitivity to dairy, cauliflower, chicken, gluten, and peas.** Other tests showed I had poor gut health and gut inflammation. The holistic doctor recommended I avoid these foods for 6 months or longer.

Also, at the recommendation of the holistic doctor, my mother made an appointment to see an allergist (a type of medical doctor) to investigate the possibility that allergies set off an attack on my body, by my body. Little did I know this visit would shed light on a multitude of dietary restrictions that would significantly impact my life.

When I entered the allergist's office, I was curious and apprehensive at the same time. I was uncomfortable with the clinic's smell. It smelled like antiseptic spray, which I hate. I could almost do nothing except think of the smell of antiseptic. The sight of medical equipment also made me nervous, but I had faith the doctor would make me feel better. Sitting in the examination room, I saw as the doctor set up several tests to find out if I had any allergies.

The findings of food sensitivity tests, blood tests, and several skin prick tests showed I'm allergic to soy, wheat, dairy, corn, and peas. This was shocking as we hadn't planned on me having such a big list of allergies.

---

[1] Hedy Marks, Medically Reviewed by Poonam Sachdev, MD, "What Is Holistic Medicine and How Does It Work?", WebMD, November 16, 2023, https://www.webmd.com/balance/what-is-holistic-medicine

The allergy doctor explained some of the test results might be false, and I might not be allergic to everything the skin prick tests showed. "About 50-60 percent of all blood tests and skin prick tests will yield a "false positive" result."[1]

Soy Sauce

I often wondered what triggered ulcerative colitis in me. Having been tested as being allergic to soy, I think having too much soy possibly caused my body to attack itself. I can't help but wonder what role soy may have played in me getting sick.

Me, dad and mom had a tradition where we would eat at a sushi restaurant every Friday. I would always eat shrimp tempura rolls (cooked fried shrimp versus raw fish), and I would drown it in soy sauce. When I say drown, I mean drown! I would dip my sushi in soy sauce, letting the rice soak up as much soy sauce as possible. The more soy sauce I could get in my body, the happier I was.

My dad would get upset and say things like, "chill out man, there's way too much salt in that." And "dude, you might as well take the top off of the soy sauce bottle, and just drink the whole bottle!"

If not for my dad's harassment, I'd likely have engulfed 3 to 5 times the amount of soy sauce I took in. I think drowning my sushi in soy sauce, combined with the heavy carbs is what caused my body to react violently and

---

[1] "Blood Tests," FARE (Food Allergy Research & Education), accessed online April 10, 2024,
https://www.foodallergy.org/resources/blood-tests

sparked my immune system to attack my body, causing my intense symptoms of ulcerative colitis to appear.

After finding out I had allergies, my father asked my mother, "why don't all kids get tested for allergies before allergies make them sick?"

My mother explained it's probably due to the high false positive rate. Whenever I have children, I plan on getting them tested early on for potential allergies, even if medical insurance won't cover the cost.

A new life

With so many allergies, how would I navigate social gatherings and school lunches? Would I have to give up my favorite foods forever? The thought of living without pizza, macaroni and cheese, and chicken nuggets left me feeling sad.

However, after the initial shock, it was time to regroup and focus on improving my health, and I knew mom and dad would support me through my journey to good health. Armed with knowledge of my allergies, we set out on a mission to transform my eating habits and way of life.

Chapter 6
The Specific Carbohydrate Diet

My mom remained depressed about my ulcerative colitis diagnosis and dove deeper into her research on autoimmune diseases and UC. About a month after my diagnosis, mommy found out about the specific carbohydrate diet (SCD) and its potential benefits for those with ulcerative colitis. She read that many people saw health improvements after switching to the diet. Also, many people on the diet were able to decrease or get rid of their ulcerative colitis symptoms and decrease or stop taking medication.

    In some cases, as people healed, they were able to expand their diet to include many of the foods they love, foods that previously made them sick. Mommy was realistic yet optimistic about the potential of the diet in helping me. Mom suggested we change my diet to see if we can further improve my health. The thought of not being sick anymore got me excited.

The specific carbohydrate diet is very restrictive and doesn't allow many foods kids love.

My mom spoke with my gastro doc about the specific carbohydrate diet. He told her he had one patient on the diet who was doing so well, he was no longer taking any medication. My doctor said the patient's mom was making a variety of SCD compliant food recipes for her son, including cakes, cookies, muffins and yogurt. He also said the patient was an athlete, which got me excited.

"The specific carbohydrate diet (SCD) is a nutritionally complete grain-free diet, low in sugar and lactose. It was developed by Dr. Sidney Haas, a pediatrician, in the 1920's as treatment for celiac disease. In 1987, Elaine Gottschall published *Breaking the Vicious Cycle*, after her daughter's inflammatory bowel disease (IBD) improved with use of the SCD." [1]

My gastro doc was concerned I may not be able to stick to the diet, because of the restrictions.

"Medical experts are still researching how this diet helps. It may be that people with certain digestive disorders are unable to break down some carbohydrates. As a result,

---

[1] "The Specific Carbohydrate Diet," Stanford Medicine, accessed online February 5, 2024.
https://med.stanford.edu/content/dam/sm/gastroenterology/documents/IBD/CarbDiet%20PDF%20final.pdf

undigested food particles stay in the intestines where bacteria grow and feed on them. This can lead to an overgrowth of harmful bacteria that irritates the intestines, which may lead to worsened gut symptoms and inflammation." [1]

As I learned more about the specific carbohydrate diet, I found it interesting that I never liked bread because it made me feel bad. It didn't hurt my tummy or get me really sick, but I just didn't feel good after eating it. Maybe my body knew all along that bread wasn't good for me.

Following the specific carbohydrate diet means you must pay attention to what's in your food and how you cook it. Since I have lots of allergies, I have to do this anyway. The SCD promotes foods that don't make me sick. I can eat fresh vegetables, meats, eggs, nuts, and some dairy products like homemade yogurt.

It can be totally tricky sometimes, reading ingredient labels and making sure you're prepping meals the right way. But, hey, if you stick with it and get the hang of things, this diet can seriously help a ton of people feel better and deal with their IBD symptoms.

Dedication

A change in diet is difficult, but it's all about being dedicated and having the right guidance to navigate through

---

[1] "Specific Carbohydrate Diet (SCD)" Cleveland Clinic, Last reviewed by a Cleveland Clinic medical professional on 07/19/2022, Copyright© 2024. accessed February 5, 2024.
https://my.clevelandclinic.org/health/treatments/23543-scd-specific-carbohydrate-diet

it all. And trust me, once I started feeling better, it was totally worth all the effort!

How I Started the Specific Carbohydrate Diet

First, my parents had a long discussion with my gastro doc and got his approval to start the diet. Also, my mom read a lot about proper nutrition, especially for those with digestive disorders. It was helpful to understand which foods are acceptable and which should be avoided when starting the specific carbohydrate diet. Mom, Dad, Nana and Gramps (my grandparents) familiarized themselves with the concepts in Elaine Gottschall's book, *Breaking The Vicious Cycle,* [1] as well as those found in other reliable sources. Then, they taught me what I needed to know about the diet.

I started the specific carbohydrate diet slowly to allow my body time to adjust to the new eating plan. A way to start SCD is to remove items that are prohibited first, and then gradually increase your consumption of foods that are allowed. Keeping a food journal helped me monitor symptoms of IBD and identify foods that triggered the symptoms. This helped me avoid bad foods in the future.

My mom made a food journal for me, keeping track of everything I ate. She also kept a poop journal, documenting whether my poop was bloody or had mucus in it. She kept this journal for more than a year.

---

[1] Elaine Gottschall B.A., M.Sc., *Breaking the Vicious Cycle, Intestinal Health Through Diet*, (Baltimore, Ontario, Canada: Kirkton Press, Fifteenth Printing, December 2014).

Skinless and Cooked Fruit

The book *Breaking The Vicious Cycle* gives guidelines that need to be followed when starting the diet. Based on what my mom read, when I started the SCD, I couldn't eat the skin on fruit, and any fruit I ate had to be cooked. So, in order to eat apples, my mom would peel and cook them. The fruit didn't have to be hot, it just had to be cooked before I ate it. So cooked fruit could be stored in the refrigerator before I ate it.

I couldn't have grapes or blueberries, because they're too small and difficult to peel. Cooked pineapples tasted strange but were still good. The diet required a lot of time and effort. I was only ten years old, so my parents and grandparents really did everything.

It was several months before I could eat blueberries or grapes, so I focused on what I could have. My grandmother would cook pineapples and mom would add honey to them to make pineapple popsicles. These are so good. To this day, they're one of my favorite treats.

Probiotics for Gut Health

When I was diagnosed with ulcerative colitis, my gastro doc told my parents I should take a probiotic called VSL3 once per day. Probiotics are live microorganisms, often referred to as "good bacteria." Since my gut health was bad, it was important for me to take a probiotic.

Adding stuff like sauerkraut and homemade yogurt, which have been fermented, can give one the good probiotics a gut needs to stay healthy. Plus, if you've got IBD like me, lots of doctors suggest taking probiotics daily to keep your gut in check. Personally, I swear by VSL3 because it works well for me.

Some people suggest not to use a probiotic pill or powder, but it's hard for me to eat that much food with probiotics in it. So, I make sure I take VSL3 daily. I usually make a smoothie with fruit and mix the VSL3 probiotic in it. Because I take a probiotic daily, I definitely didn't follow the exact rules specified in some literature on the specific carbohydrate diet, but the small tweaks I made worked for me and I saw major health improvements.

Not everyone is a good candidate

Although many people's digestive health has greatly improved as a result of the specific carbohydrate diet, it's crucial to understand that not everyone is a good candidate for it. Certain food groups may be too restrictive for some people to follow, or they may find it difficult to consume enough when following the dietary restrictions.

A strong commitment is needed for the SCD to work, which can be challenging when eating out or in social settings. To handle these situations, one must be able to prepare ahead, explain dietary needs to others (like to a waiter at a restaurant), and defend oneself by avoiding foods not compliant with the SCD, as well as foods one is allergic to.

Dietary Deficiencies and Side Effects

I needed a lot of support, and I got it from my

parents, grandparents, doctors and friends. It was crucial that my parents, grandparents and doctors monitored for any signs of dietary deficiencies or unfavorable side effects while following the SCD and dealing with my ulcerative colitis.

Working closely with my healthcare providers to find and address any potential issues helped ensure my nutritional needs were met, and digestive problems were appropriately controlled. I meet with my pediatrician and gastro doc several times a year, at minimum.

My weight was checked carefully. My gastro doc was concerned that it would be hard for me to gain weight. I was already underweight and when I got sick, I lost weight.

I HAD TO ELIMINATE SUGAR

One thing forbidden on the specific carbohydrate is processed sugar. This is extremely difficult because so many people are addicted to sugar. And sugar is in so many foods people commonly eat, often disguised as "high fructose corn syrup." My dad told me he'd have a lot of trouble cutting sugar from his diet, because he is so used to eating things that are full of sugar.

So, what do I do for birthday parties, or gatherings? They'll definitely be serving pizza, ice cream and cake. Will I have to skip parties and gatherings? The next 5-6 months on the specific carbohydrate diet were really hard.

I had to drop sugar from my diet! I could have eased my way off of sugar by decreasing the number of sugary foods and snacks I was used to eating. However, I stopped eating anything with processed sugar in it as soon as I learned this rule about the specific carbohydrate diet.

The bad thing is, a short time after I started the diet, I started cheating and didn't tell my parents.

My parents told me not to eat anything at school other than the food they packed for me. But I felt bad watching other kids eat cookies at my afterschool program. I wanted to eat the cookies too. I loved those cookies.

They had yummy cream filled cookies at my afterschool program. Every chance I got, I'd gobble down some cookies. I'd break the cookies apart by separating the top and bottom, then I'd either lick the cream filled center, or I'd scrape the tasty center off with my teeth and savor the taste. Then I'd eat the rest of the cookie. If I could have grabbed a whole box of those cookies without anyone catching me, I'd have snuck to where no one could see me and eaten the whole box. Those cookies were good!

But I felt bloated after eating the cookies. They literally made me sick. My stomach would hurt bad. Yet, I continued to eat the cookies after school. But after dealing with a couple of flare-ups, some of them bad, I decided to avoid the cookies. My options were eat the cookies and be sick, or stick to the specific carbohydrate diet and have a chance of being healthy.

This was a turning point for me, but I cheated on the specific carbohydrate diet again, this time with my parents' permission, as I'll explain. I could clearly see why my gastro doc thought I'd have a hard time doing this diet. He was right!

How we knew for sure The Specific Carbohydrate Diet works for me

While strictly following the specific carbohydrate diet for over a month after I stopped eating cookies, my UC symptoms stopped. I was still taking the Canasa medication and didn't feel great, but at least I didn't feel sick, my stomach didn't hurt, and my poop was normal. When my school's spring break came, my family traveled out of town. Mom and dad decided I could eat anything I wanted, and I did. Within a few days of eating food that the SCD prohibits, I had a flare-up. I got sicker by the end of spring break and was sick into the next week. My stomach was killing me. I also had blood and mucus in my poop, as well as diarrhea. This was terrible!

My parents felt guilty for allowing me to eat whatever I wanted while on vacation.

Getting sick on vacation was another turning point for me. Me and my parents were so sad when I got sick. When we returned home, I started the specific carbohydrate diet again from scratch.

Like many kids, I ate candy before being diagnosed with ulcerative colitis, but my parents always stopped me from eating what they considered too much. While on spring break I ate sugary foods but didn't eat a lot and still got sick.

MY RESILIENT WIN

It became clear my body has a tough time handing sugar and refined carbohydrates like cookies, cakes, candies, white rice, sugary drinks, bread and cereals.

"Eating too much added sugar and other refined carbs is linked to inflammation in the body — which may lead to health problems. But eating more fiber may be a powerful way to reduce inflammation, with other lifestyle changes."[1]

After I stopped cheating on the diet by eating cookies and the foods I ate while on spring break, I haven't knowingly eaten any foods with processed sugar in them since then. Also, I haven't eaten any processed food since then. I now only eat "real food" with wholesome ingredients. Newer studies completed a few years after my diagnosis "found evidence that added sugar in the diet can lead to IBD, and also make existing disease worse."[2]

No Medications

After I stopped cheating on the specific carbohydrate diet, after several more months, I showed no

---

[1] Mary Jane Brown, PhD, RD, medically reviewed by Adam Bernstein, MD, ScD, "Does Sugar Cause Inflammation in the Body?," Healthline, updated on February 26, 2024, accessed online April 10, 2024, https://www.healthline.com/nutrition/sugar-and-inflammation

[2] Eve M. Glazier, MD, and Elizabeth Ko, MD, "Initial Studies link added sugar and IBD," UCLA Health, February 26, 2021, https://www.uclahealth.org/news/initial-studies-link-added-sugar-and-ibd

The Specific Carbohydrate Diet

symptoms of ulcerative colitis. My gastro doc had me take some tests for inflammation markers, and the tests came back negative, meaning they didn't show any signs of ulcerative colitis. So, I was allowed to stop taking any prescription medication for ulcerative colitis.

I stayed symptom free from inflammatory bowel disease after I stopped taking medication. But after a few weeks on no meds, minor symptoms of ulcerative colitis did reoccur. These instances were considered flare-ups, and usually disappeared within a few days.

Based on the body of knowledge known about the specific carbohydrate diet, periodic flare-ups, where symptoms of IBD reappear are common. "An ulcerative colitis flare-up is the return of symptoms after not having any for a period of time. This may involve diarrhea, belly pain and cramping, rectal pain and bleeding, fatigue, and urgent bowel movements." [1]

Over the next few months, I had several more flare-ups. Some of the flare-ups were bad enough, my mom called my gastro doc for advice. In some cases, my gastro doc recommended I take my Canasa prescription for a few days to help control my IBD symptoms, then once the symptoms disappeared, I could stop taking the medication again and see what happens. I followed my doctor's recommendation.

My flare-ups included mucus in my poop and stomach pain, and sometimes some blood in my poop. After 5 or 6 flare-ups, the flare-ups stopped. **Within three**

---

[1] Ulcerative colitis flare-ups: 5 tips to manage them, July 19, 2023. The Mayo Clinic. https://www.mayoclinic.org/diseases-conditions/ulcerative-colitis/in-depth/ulcerative-colitis-flare-up/art-20120410

years after starting the specific carbohydrate diet and following it strictly, I stopped having any IBD symptoms and I've not had any symptoms since.

One thing that happens to me sometimes is if I eat food I'm allergic to by accident, I break out in hives. When this occurs, I've always taken over the counter Zyrtec 10 mg allergy relief dissolvable tabs. The itching and redness on my skin due to hives usually goes away in 24 hours or less.

Adjusting to the SCD and reintroducing some foods

With the specific carbohydrate diet, I'm able to avoid foods I'm allergic to and eliminate the symptoms of IBD. Honey completely replaced processed sugar, so I still enjoy sweet tasting food. And since I don't eat processed food, I don't get exposed to many of the things that made me sick.

I felt a range of emotions as I got used to my new eating limitations with allergies, and the many great things I could eat while on the SCD. I had triumphant moments when I tried new meals and tastes, as well as frustrating ones when I missed the foods I used to love. I developed the ability to analyze food labels and avoid things I'm allergic to. I also had to maintain the discipline to avoid peer pressure when at social gatherings, so I wouldn't eat foods my body can't handle.

Despite the difficulties, having IBD helped me experience great life changes. I started paying more attention to my health and well-being and gave my body the nutritious meals it needed. People who I let know about my allergies become considerate and aware of my food requirements.

Rather than being a burden, ulcerative colitis gave me power. I accepted my special dietary needs with courage and hope, knowing that the trade-offs were good for my health. I flourished thanks to the love and support of my family, friends, and medical team, showing that allergies and UC were not barriers to growth but rather chances for personal development.

I gained vital knowledge about resiliency, and self-care from my experiences with inflammatory bowel disease. What started off as a trip to the doctor turned into a life-changing event that changed my perspective on everything. I became stronger and more independent as I learned to deal with the highs and lows of having ulcerative colitis. I was prepared to take on any obstacles that came my way.

We confirmed earlier food sensitivity and allergy tests, proving I'm allergic to soy, wheat, dairy, corn, and peas.

Since some of the skin prick tests for allergies could have been false positive results, based on my allergy doctor's recommendation, after 6 months, we slowly phased some of the foods I tested as allergic to back into my diet. This was done only after my symptoms of ulcerative colitis disappeared. We also phased in foods I tested as sensitive to, based on my holistic doctor's recommendation, making sure there was coordination between what all my doctors thought. After a year, we phased chicken back into my diet. Yes! I Love Chicken!

Another great benefit of the specific carbohydrate diet for me is the increased power of my mind!

The immediate impact of cutting sugar from my diet is I went from being an okay student to an elite student. This change happened overnight, helping me graduate as the top ranked student academically at my middle school. When I used to be high on sugar much of the time, I couldn't sit still and focus. Suddenly, with zero sugar or processed food in my diet, it was easy for me to focus. Also, a few months after starting the specific carbohydrate diet, my body was able handle eating fresh, uncooked blueberries, grapes, and pineapples, but I still avoided uncooked apples. Also, I made sure I didn't eat too much uncooked fruit.

In summary

The specific carbohydrate diet emphasizes dietary modifications that lessen symptoms of digestive disorders and improve gut health. Implementing the SCD requires perseverance and dedication, but many people who use it have reported a decrease or elimination of their symptoms and an improvement in their quality of life. If people understand the principles of the SCD, plan their meals thoughtfully, and get the help they need, they can successfully follow it and reap its potential benefits for their digestive health.

Typical foods that are allowed on the SCD are:

1. Fresh fruit (not processed or canned).
2. Vegetables (of the non-starchy variety).
3. Seeds and nuts, but in moderation (once symptoms of IBD are gone for a while).
4. Legumes (once soaked and allowed to sprout).
5. Seafood and meat.
6. Organic aged cheeses (without additives).
7. To eliminate lactose, homemade yogurt is fermented for a full day.

Foods to avoid:

1. Cereals and grains.
2. Foods processed and having preservatives or additions.
3. Carbohydrate-rich veggies, like potatoes.
4. Most dairy products (apart from homemade yogurt and aged cheeses).
5. Most syrups, artificial sweeteners, and refined sugars.
6. Processed and canned fruits.

Chapter 7
Meal Planning

Meal planning is super important when you're doing the specific carbohydrate diet. You wanna make sure you're getting the best nutrition and managing your IBD symptoms well. You gotta plan your meals carefully. That means knowing what you can and can't eat. My parents got me involved in planning and preparing my meals, so it won't be a shock to me when I go off to college. I try out different recipes and mix things up to keep my diet interesting while still sticking to the rules.

I don't think there is a one size fit all approach to being on the SCD, but there are some rules I followed.

MY RESILIENT WIN

SCD meal preparation

1. Consultation with a healthcare provider

If you have inflammatory bowel disease, it's important to see a healthcare professional before changing your diet. A gastroenterologist and registered dietitian experienced in treating inflammatory bowel illnesses are great choices. To guarantee effectiveness and safety, they may check your progress and provide tailored suggestions. My doctor watched my weight carefully.

2. Understanding what you can and can't eat

Become acquainted with the specific carbohydrate diet's list of permitted and prohibited foods. Fresh fruits, non-starchy vegetables, meats, seafood, eggs, certain nuts, and homemade yogurt are usually considered permissible foods. Grains, sugary sweets, most dairy products, processed foods, and additives are examples of restricted foods.

3. Creating Balanced Meals

Arrange meals so there's a good mix of protein, good fats, fruits and specific carbohydrates that are safe to eat (many vegetables fit in this category). I like lean meats like chicken and fish, but occasionally eat beef and pork. I also like veggies like broccoli, string beans, asparagus, carrots, and spinach. I include healthy fats to help me feel full and help vitamins get in my body, like nuts, avocados, and olive oil.

4. Using different recipes for variety

Preparing meals in different and creative ways using permitted items. This includes stir-fried vegetables, grilled fish with lemon and herbs, and homemade chicken soup with veggies and bone broth. Instead of using premade sauces or seasonings, try adding flavor using herbs and spices.

5. Managing meal preparation

Since preparing meals on the specific carbohydrate diet takes much more time than buying fast food or heating processed frozen food in a microwave oven, the diet is hard to follow. But meal preparation can be simplified by making multiple meals at the same time and saving prepared meals for later.

Choosing a day to make basic dishes like grilled chicken breasts and roasted vegetables is a great idea. This reduces stress and saves time. Instead of cooking every meal from scratch, my family simply stores and reheats cooked meals when I'm ready to eat them during the week.

6. Tracking symptoms and adjusting

My mom keeps a food journal to record meals, noting any association between certain foods and getting sick. A smart phone makes this easier to do. To reduce IBD symptoms and encourage recovery, I keep aware of possible trigger foods and modify my diet to avoid them. Under my doctor's supervision, I thought about gradually reintroducing limited foods to gauge my body's reaction to them.

MY RESILIENT WIN

7. Prioritizing gut health

I made gut health a priority and take probiotics daily. In addition to following the specific carbohydrate diet, I stay well hydrated by drinking enough water. I also focus on controlling my stress levels and getting enough sleep to help my body recover and/or stay healthy. As part of the SCD, I include foods high in probiotics like fermented veggies or homemade yogurt. These lifestyle choices are essential for me in maintaining healthy digestion and general wellbeing.

REMEMBER: MY MOM LOST HER HEARING IN ONE EAR, POSSIBLY DUE TO STRESS.

Some meal samples for the specific carbohydrate diet

Breakfasts:

- Scrambled eggs with sautéed spinach, scrambled in avocado oil.
- Almond flour pancakes with sliced bananas, blueberries or strawberries, with honey on top instead of syrup.
- Homemade yogurt topped with chopped almonds and fresh fruit.
- Hard boiled eggs with sea salt.

Lunches:

- Grilled chicken breast with broccoli.
- Grilled chicken salad with olive oil vinaigrette dressing.
- Hamburgers wrapped in lettuce instead of bread (or with lettuce and tomatoes on the side).

Dinners:

- Baked salmon with roasted asparagus.
- Stir fried beef with bell peppers and broccoli.
- Zucchini noodles with homemade marinara sauce and ground turkey or beef.

Snacks:

- Fresh fruit or dried fruits.
- Almond butter on sliced apples.
- Carrot sticks.
- Homemade yogurt.
- Almonds.

Meal planning is totally key to keeping IBD symptoms under control and helping you recover. The focus is eating unprocessed foods and eliminating complex carbs. This can really do wonders for your gut health, inflammation levels, and overall well-being.

MY RESILIENT WIN

It's super important to talk with a healthcare provider to make sure a diet is safe for you. With careful planning and a bit of experimenting, you can still enjoy delicious, nutritious meals while managing IBD symptoms and living your best life.

Chapter 8
Butternut Squash Fries

I love French fries! I love them so much I would eat them for every meal if I could, even for breakfast. I love to drown crispy French fries in ketchup and eat them until I'm stuffed. Sometimes, when I sleep, I dream of eating French fries. But to follow the specific carbohydrate diet, I had to stop eating French fries because they made me sick. Also, most ketchup is loaded with sugar, so is also non-compliant for me.

My mom found a great swap for potato French fries: butternut squash fries with honey-based ketchup! Seriously, these fries are the bomb, and I've never even missed the potato ones. They're super tasty and way healthier too, especially when you dip them in honey-based ketchup. It's like the perfect combo!

MY RESILIENT WIN

Preparing butternut squash fries

My mom, dad or nana (grandmother) buy fresh butternut squash, peel them, remove the seed filled center, and cut them into the shape of French fries. To cook butternut squash fries to perfection, my mom, dad and nana use one of three methods:

1. Bake in an oven.
2. Fry on a stovetop.
3. Crisp in an air-fryer.

Oven baked butternut squash

1. Pre-heat oven to 400 degrees.
2. Place parchment paper on a baking sheet, then evenly distribute the sliced butternut squash on top of the parchment paper.
3. Lightly cover with avocado oil (or spray with avocado oil).

Since I'm allergic to corn and soy, my family cooking team can't use corn or soy oil and prefers avocado oil over canola oil because of its antioxidants.

4. Add some sea salt (but not too much).
5. Once the temperature reaches 400 degrees, place baking sheet on the center oven rack and bake for 10 minutes.
6. Remove the baking sheet, flip the butternut squash fries, add a little more avocado oil and salt.
7. Return the butternut squash fries to oven and bake for an added 10 to 12 minutes or until crispy.

8. Remove from oven, let sit for two minutes (or when cool enough to eat).

Depending on how moist the butternut squash is, the butternut squash should be crispy. Since the texture of butternut squash varies much more than a potato, some of the butternut squash fries might be less crispy, but still taste extremely good.

Fried butternut squash

1. Use a deep pan to pre-heat cooking oil on medium to high heat. My family cooking team typically fill a pan with about ¼ of an inch of avocado oil (using avocado oil as explained previously). Once the oil is hot, add the cut butternut squash fries, being careful not to let the oil splash on you.
2. To avoid getting splashed by oil, for safety, use 12–18-inch tongs to gently place the butternut squash fries into the hot oil and avoid making a splash.
3. Cook covered or uncovered and adjust the heat as needed. Cook until crispy (usually between 10-12 minutes).
4. Remove the fries from the pan and place them on a plate covered with a paper towel (to soak up excess oil), add salt as desired.
5. Let sit for at least 2 minutes (or until cool enough to eat).

MY RESILIENT WIN

Air fried butternut squash

Follow the specific instructions on one's air fryer for cooking French fries. Many air fryers have an "air crisp" function, which is what my family cooking team uses on a Ninja Grill brand air fryer.

1. Place the butternut squash fries in the air fryer basket.
2. Lightly cover or spray with the oil of your choice.

In my case avocado oil.

3. Add salt as desired.
4. Cook for 10 minutes, turn fries over.
5. Cook for an additional 10-12 minutes or until crispy.
6. Remove from air frier and let sit for at least 2 minutes (or until cool enough to eat).

Sometimes my family cooking team uses extra virgin olive oil instead of avocado oil and it creates an extra nice flavor. But some professional chefs claim the health benefits of olive oil are decreased if olive oil is subjected to high heat. Also, many professional chefs claim avocado oil burns better and is more ideal for cooking at high temperatures.

My ketchup dilemma

Since most ketchup has lots of sugar in it and can trigger symptoms of IBD, I use Wellbee's honey sweetened ketchup. It's all natural with no sugar added. It's also paleo and SCD friendly. My mother orders the ketchup directly from Wellbee's or Amazon.com. When we travel, I always bring Wellbee's ketchup and barbecue sauce with me.

The link for Wellbee's ketchup:
https://www.wellbees.com/ketchup.html

I completely fill my desire for French fries with ketchup by eating butternut squash fries and using Wellbee's ketchup. I eat butternut squash fries several times per week and don't miss potato French fries at all.

When friends came to my house, they tried butternut squash fries and liked them!

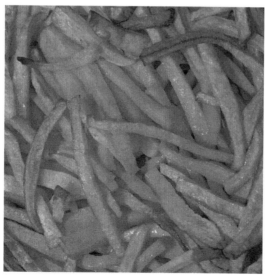

Butternut squash fries

Chapter 9
Dining Out

At times I have to eat at restaurants, especially when I travel. For people with inflammatory bowel disease, eating out can be difficult. This is extra challenging in my case, because in addition to being on the specific carbohydrate diet, as I've said, I also have several allergies. The last thing I want to do is eat something that makes me sick.

The first thing I avoid when traveling is eating at fast-food restaurants. While fast food can be convenient, much of it can make me sick. Fast food is cheap compared to most full-service restaurants, but I often have to pay extra money for the sake of my health. The only fast-food restaurant I commonly eat at is Five Guys. This is because many fast-food restaurants use ingredients, even in hamburgers, that I can't eat, like soy protein as a filler. As always, I avoid soy, gluten and dairy, so I don't eat bread with a burger at Five Guys restaurant.

MY RESILIENT WIN

Planning

I have to plan my meals when dining out. Since I can't eat ketchup or barbeque sauce with processed sugar in it, I travel with my honey-based ketchup and barbeque sauce. With hamburgers, I like ketchup, but if I'm having chicken, steak or lamb, I like barbeque sauce. So, when I fly somewhere out of town, I pack several bottles of each in my checked luggage, always making sure I have enough for the entire trip.

When I'm going out to eat, depending on what I plan to eat, I'll bring a bottle of ketchup or barbecue sauce with me in a backpack. If I'm not sure which one I'll have, I'll bring both. If for some reason I don't have my special ketchup or barbeque sauce with me, I either have no sauce at all or use mustard. As long as the mustard doesn't have additional additives like sugar or corn syrup, my body can tolerate it.

To comply with my dietary needs, me and my parents research restaurants before we travel. We'll select from among many depending on what we're in the mood to eat. My mom often calls restaurants ahead of time to verify how they prepare food and if any of the ingredients might make me sick.

When at a restaurant, I let my server know about my allergies to help avoid eating anything that might make me sick. Waiters are human, so they can make mistakes. If for some reason the people at a restaurant aren't sure of the ingredients of a dish I'm considering eating, I choose something else to eat, and possibly go to a different restaurant.

Dining Out

My advice for eating out while following the specific carbohydrate diet:

1. Do advance research on restaurants

Find out whether restaurants can handle your dietary restrictions or provide alternative choices not on the menu before heading out to eat. Look for menus that provide personalized alternatives along with wholesome foods.

2. Explain your dietary needs

Let the restaurant staff know about your dietary needs when you make reservations or when you arrive. Explain the things you can't eat, and ask about any possible changes to their menu, or replacements to help you stay safe.

3. Focus on eating simple, unprocessed foods

Make menu selections that include approved SCD items such grilled meats, seafood, eggs, and non-starchy veggies. Avoid foods with processed sugars and grains.

4. Request menu modifications

Don't be afraid to ask for changes in how your food is made that the restaurant doesn't have on the menu. It's your health, and you deserve special treatment to meet your dietary needs. For instance, I've gone to diners and asked if

MY RESILIENT WIN

I can have eggs scrambled in avocado oil, olive oil or ghee if possible, so I can avoid butter. If a restaurant can't accommodate me, then I'll ask for hardboiled eggs, even if it's not on the menu. I request steamed or grilled vegetables instead of rice or potatoes as a side dish. And I ask for a hamburger wrapped in lettuce, versus served on a bun. I avoid dressings and sauces.

5. Pay attention to hidden ingredients

Seasonings, marinades, and sauces are examples of hidden ingredients that may include non-compliant carbs. To make sure the food complies with the SCD, ask to see ingredient lists or have a conversation with the chef if possible. It's often important to ask to speak to the chef, as some restaurant staff might not understand that certain sauces might be loaded with sugar, corn syrup, or soy, so be careful.

6. Make plans for social events

If you're going to eat out with friends or attend a social event, make advanced plans by recommending restaurants that provide SCD-friendly menu items, or eat in advance and don't eat at the event. Possibly, only have a snack at the event. I've attended many catered events where I've asked for a special meal, and the caterer was able to provide one for me.

What I do at birthday parties is I bring my own cupcakes. My mom will make cupcakes for me the night before that have tasty, honey-based frosting. She'll put them in Tupperware for me and when everyone else gets cake and starts to eat it, I eat my special cupcakes. This is not as big of an issue now that I'm older, but it was important to me when I was ten.

7. Pack safe snacks and bring any special condiments

If there aren't many alternatives, bring snacks that are safe for you to eat like fresh fruit or other safe snacks. You won't starve and you'll stay safe. Also, if you have special ketchup or barbeque sauce, make sure to bring it.

If I'm going to a movie theater that doesn't allow people to bring in food, I carry a letter from my doctor that explains my dietary requirements and will show it to the theater manager if necessary.

8. Limit eating out

While you can often find good food choices when eating out, it's still possible to get exposed to foods that aren't safe for you. And if you give into temptation and eat something you know might make you sick, try to limit how much of an unapproved food you eat. This will help limit any possible IBD symptoms. To help with digestion, eating smaller, frequent meals might help.

9. Remain hydrated

Staying well hydrated may help you in digesting food and give you a feeling of fullness. This can help you avoid overeating any non-compliant foods.

10. Listen to your body

Pay attention to the impact of different meals and dining scenarios on your body. If you have discomfort or IBD symptoms after eating something, make a note of it to avoid selecting that dish in the future. This approach can help you make smart eating choices that help keep you from getting sick.

Careful preparation, open communication, and flexibility are necessary while eating and adhering to the specific carbohydrate diet for those with inflammatory bowel disease. People with IBD can handle social events while following the SCD guidelines by doing their homework on restaurants, stating their dietary preferences, and making thoughtful decisions. For those with IBD, eating out can be a fun activity that promotes social and physical well-being when done with the right planning and understanding.

11. Worst Case Scenario (be prepared)

As part of my planning, when I travel on vacation, especially internationally, I plan for the worst-case scenario, the possibility I have a flare-up. I always bring a Prednisone and Canasa prescription with me. This was recommended by my pediatric gastroenterologist. Though I've never had a flare-up on vacation since I stopped taking medication for ulcerative colitis, it's a good idea to have medication with me. Note, Prednisone is supposed to work faster than Canasa in fighting inflammation.

Chapter 10

Managing Food Cravings

Anyone with inflammatory bowel disease faces lots of challenges. Trying to stick with the specific carbohydrate can also be challenging. Imagine what I think when I see a kid eating candy or cookies. Remember, when I first started the specific carbohydrate diet, I ate cookies, even though I knew they were bad for me. I craved those cookies.

Most people like candy, I know I do. Each day at school, I see kids eating candy. I definitely want some, but I know I can't eat it. I'm in a battle for good health. Yes, I want candy, but I have to fight the urge and manage cravings. I remember how bad it feels to have a flare-up. This memory helps me avoid these cravings.

Pressure

There is pressure to eat bad food everywhere. We see it in commercials where people are laughing, dancing and having fun. Psychologically, this makes me want to laugh, dance and have fun too. But like I said, I'm in a battle for good health. I've never seen a commercial where people are eating grilled salmon and broccoli while laughing, dancing and having fun. But eating healthy has become fun for me.

People celebrate with ice cream and cake. I used to love ice cream, but as I write this book, I'm 17 years old and haven't had ice cream in 7 years. I know my daddy eats ice cream, but thankfully, he avoids eating things I can't eat while in my presence. The same goes for mom. I'm in a battle for good health, and if you want good health, it's worth the fight.

Social Pressures

Schools, parties, and other get-togethers where unhealthy foods are served can cause some to eat foods they shouldn't eat. Often, people will insist you eat foods that can make you sick, and you might give into social pressures. If you don't eat the bad foods, frustration and feelings of loneliness may result. But if you eat bad foods, you may have an IBD flare-up. You also might be overcome by feelings of guilt, after eating bad foods.

To avoid feeling sad when I see people eating foods I love but can't eat anymore, I bring my own treats. This includes SCD approved honey-based candy and my special cupcakes made with almond flour.

Cravings and Temptations

People, but especially kids, may find it difficult to follow any type of diet restrictions. While friends and family are enjoying eating unhealthy foods in front of you, it's easy to crave processed foods, candy, and other things that are off-limits. I must deal with this often.

I went to a sporting event and there were two people right in front of me who were eating cotton candy like it was the best sugar laden substance ever created. They literally kept talking about how great the cotton candy was. To make matters worse, they were making loud noises emphasizing how much they were enjoying the cotton cady. It's hard to describe my emotions, but I used to love cotton candy. I certainly wanted some, but the thought of getting sick helped me control my emotions.

Limited Food Options

Due to the SCD's restrictions, there may be few options for food at times, which may make meals dull and disappointing. You might get tired of eating many of the same foods on the specific carbohydrate diet.

Emotional Impact

Children who live with a chronic illness such as ulcerative colitis may experience emotional strain, which may intensify cravings and temptations as a coping strategy. My dad is a stress eater. When he gets stressed out, he'll eat the worst foods for him, and a ton of it. There are lots of people who do this. If this is you, it's a good idea to find a better way to manage stress than eating bad foods. Seeking help from a psychology professional may be helpful. For me, I like to exercise to help manage my stress.

My dad told me when he was about ten years old, his mother bought a coffee cake and put it in the refrigerator. He saw the coffee cake and decided to eat a slice. Well, things didn't go as planned because he ended up eating the entire cake.

"Man," my dad said, "my mother kicked my butt!"

I don't know why my dad ate the entire coffee cake. Perhaps it would have been better not to eat a slice at all. But he craved the coffee cake so much that despite knowing he was going to catch an old school 1970s beatdown, he decided a brutal beatdown was worth eating the entire coffee cake. Is such reasoning justified? Emotional decisions can make matters worse.

Suppose I gave into temptation and ate a giant piece of cotton candy. While I know it would have tasted good and would have provided me with temporary enjoyment. I also know it could make me sick, similar to how my dad knew he would get in trouble. Life is full of choices, but I think the best choice is the healthiest choice.

Techniques for Handling Cravings and Temptations

Despite these difficulties, parents and loved ones may use the following tactics to help kids control cravings while on the SCD. These tips also work for adults.

1. Education about good snacks

It's critical to teach kids how certain foods affect their health, and there's always a healthy alternative to eating something that can make them sick. For instance, fresh fruit dipped in honey tastes as good or better to me than most candy. I remember dipping apple slices in almond butter and honey while kids around me ate candy, and I was just as happy. Also, there are honey-based candies that are compliant with the SCD. I usually carry multiple honey based peanut bars with me, and I eat one or two if I'm craving something sweet. The peanuts help me feel full and the honey gives me the sweet taste I like.

2. Meal planning and preparation

Getting involved in meal planning activities might help one become more excited about the specific carbohydrate diet. With kids, encourage them to go grocery shopping with you and help in choosing items to prepare later. Also, allow kids to choose the specific dishes they want to eat that follow the SCD.

3. Food substitutions

It's a good idea to plan out replacements for foods one can't eat. For instance, try making handmade SCD-friendly pastries using nut flours, honey, and fruits instead of sugary cakes and pies.

4. Reinforce positive behavior

Show your appreciation for a kid's dedication in following the SCD. Praise them and tell them something like, "you must be proud of yourself." Also, you might want to give them rewards for their dedication, like posters, stickers, books, comic books, or other rewards. A child or adult should feel empowered by the specific carbohydrate diet and should praise themselves for a job well done. This diet is not easy, but I have seen the benefits.

5. Peer support

If possible, connect with other families who are managing inflammatory bowel disease or other illnesses. Children who get peer support may feel like they fit in, and this might make it easier to handle their food restrictions.

6. Communication

Talk openly with friends, family, and teachers about a child's dietary needs and foods they can't eat. Give tips on what alternatives work and politely say no to foods that won't work for them. Special in-class treats can be a stressful time at school for kids with inflammatory bowel disease, so communicating with teachers is important.

7. Flexibility and moderation

Although managing ulcerative colitis requires careful commitment to the SCD, eating non-compliant meals may be allowed sometimes. Some people can reintroduce non-compliant foods like potatoes after long durations with no flare-ups. Stress the value of making good food choices.

8. Keep your doctor involved

This will help you avoid problems. Also, if you have a dietician, keep them involved as you manage the specific carbohydrate diet.

In summary

It might be hard to control food cravings while doing the specific carbohydrate diet, especially for kids. But encouraging kids to follow the SCD and take good care of their health is easier with a support system. Smart snacks can help people manage food cravings.

Classmates have wondered how I can keep from eating candy. For me, I remember the pain of a UC flare-up. I don't want to experience that again.

Chapter 11
Strategies for Staying Symptom Free

The symptoms of inflammatory bowel disease suck. No way do I want to deal with symptoms of ulcerative colitis. With my symptoms gone, I want to make sure I don't get them again. If they return, I will fight to get the symptoms back in remission. This might sound simple, but keeping symptoms of UC in remission can be difficult. If one can use the following strategies, the possibility of avoiding symptoms of UC is increased.

1. Stick to the specific carbohydrate diet

The diet works for me, so it's important I follow it. This means avoiding foods not allowed by checking labels when shopping and preparing foods correctly.

2. Keeping a food journal

Using a notebook, spreadsheet, or app, one can track what they've eaten. If I end up with symptoms of IBD, reviewing my journal will help me figure out what might have helped trigger my IBD symptoms.

3. Keep learning about specific carbohydrate diet

The diet can't be learned in one day. By continuing to learn about the diet, at some point, you'll probably be an expert. Knowing the specific carbohydrate diet well can help you stick to it better. There are books, websites, and groups that can give you tips and support. It's also good to talk to your doctor or a dietitian for advice.

4. Be careful with new foods

Take it easy when you start the SCD. When you start feeling better and feel ready to try raw fruit vs. cooked fruit, maybe eat small amounts of raw fruit as an addition to cooked fruit. Consult with your doctor and dietitian once your IBD symptoms are reduced or eliminated. Then, you might be able to eat some non-compliant foods.

When you're ready to introduce some of your favorite foods, try not to eat a lot of it. Along with using a food journal, being careful will help you decide which foods might be a problem, and they'll be less of a problem if you don't eat a lot of it.

5. Eat Healthy Foods

Eating foods that give you the proper nutrients your body needs is important for staying healthy. Supplements might also be helpful, but you should consult with your doctor to make sure whatever you take is safe and ideal for you. Eating healthy foods should be a nice experience.

6. Manage Stress

Stress can make an illness worse. I use an app called "Calm" on my iPhone that I heard LeBron James uses, and it helps me relax. My dad meditates which helps him relax. Adequate sleep, exercise, social activities, and relaxation can help you feel better. My mom gardens and goes for long walks. What works best for you can only be decided by you, but these are just some suggestions.

When I'm stressed out, I like to lift weights or play basketball, and this puts my mind at ease. Sometimes I just go to a local park and run. The air going into my lungs makes me feel strong and free.

7. Keep in Touch with Your Doctor

It's crucial to have regular check-ups with your doctor to manage IBD well. These appointments can help one make prompt adjustments to their treatment if needed. Support from doctors is important for the healing process. By staying in touch with your healthcare team, you improve your chance of maintaining a better quality of life, despite the challenges of having inflammatory bowel disease.

8. Personalize Your Plan

Every person with IBD is different. Your diet plan should fit your needs. Work with your healthcare team, including your doctor and dietitian, to create a plan that works best for you.

9. Have a support system

Everyone has things they have to deal with. I was determined not to let IBD define me. I had the support of my parents, grandparents, medical team and friends. My gastro doc was concerned about my weight and wondered how the diet may impact my weight. So, I had frequent appointments with my gastro doc to ensure I was healthy while on the specific carbohydrate diet. Over time, my weight began to increase, and I was no longer frail and skinny.

Conclusion

Sticking to the specific carbohydrate diet can help keep inflammatory bowel disease symptoms in check. By following these simple strategies, like sticking to the diet, eating healthy, and managing stress, you can improve your chances of staying in remission. It's important to work with your healthcare team to find the right plan for you. With dedication and support, you can manage your IBD symptoms and enjoy a better quality of life.

Chapter 12
The Importance of Exercise

In addition to my diet, exercise plays an important role in helping me manage inflammatory bowel disease. Being physically fit helps me feel good. It keeps my mind sharp because my body is strong.

When I was first diagnosed with inflammatory bowel disease, I was too sick to get much exercise. Despite being dedicated to being physically fit, I didn't have the energy to get much exercise. But after starting the specific carbohydrate diet and suppressing my IBD symptoms, I got back into the routine of exercising. I started off gradually and worked my way back into great physical condition. Now my strength and stamina are great.

I'm an athlete! I work out almost every day. I love working out. Exercising is part of who I am. I can't imagine not working out. I can't envision a period in my life where I don't work out consistently.

Exercising makes me feel good. It makes me strong. It gives me power. Exercising is worth the effort!

"If you have ulcerative colitis (UC), exercise can help you feel better and prevent some common problems that are related to the disease. Check out these great ways that workouts can boost your health. Your doctor can help you decide what kind of activity -- and how much -- is best for you.

1. Strengthen Your Bones

2. Keep Your Muscles and Joints Working

3. Recover From Surgery Faster

4. Lower Stress

5. Lift Your Mood

6. Help Prevent Colon Cancer" [1]

---

[1] Camille Peri, Medically Reviewed by Neha Pathak, MD, FACP, DipABLM on May 3, 2024, "6 Benefits of Exercise for Ulcerative Colitis," https://www.webmd.com/ibd-crohns-disease/ulcerative-colitis/uc-exercise

The Importance of Exercise

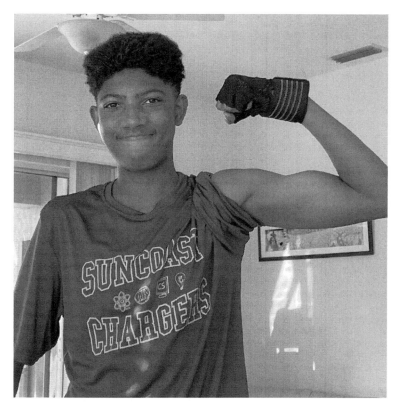

Exercising makes me feel good

MY RESILIENT WIN

Joint pain and inflammatory bowel disease

Midway through my first-year season of high school basketball, I started to have knee pain. I didn't think much of it at first, as knee pain for basketball players is common. But my knee pain got progressively worse. My parents thought I might have torn a ligament, so we consulted with my pediatrician.

It ends up: "The most common non-digestive issue for people with UC is joint pain."[1]

So, at the recommendation of my pediatrician, I met with an orthopedic surgeon. After an opinion by one surgeon, I got a second opinion from another surgeon. To the surgeons, it looked like I was having growing pains (osteochondritis dissecans), but doctors were not sure if it was related to ulcerative colitis (which was a possibility).

The first surgeon wanted to do surgery. The second surgeon wanted me to do physical therapy to get blood flowing properly in my joints, and potentially heal my knee without surgery. Healing naturally would avoid any scar tissue build up.

We also consulted with my gastroenterologist, who ordered a specific test to find out if my joint pain was due to ulcerative colitis. The test confirmed the joint pain was not due to ulcerative colitis.

---

[1] Kathryn Whitbourne, Medically Reviewed by Tyler Wheeler, MD on August 12, 2022, "Ulcerative Colitis and Join Pain," WebMD, https://www.webmd.com/ibd-crohns-disease/ulcerative-colitis/ulcerative-colitis-joint-pain

The Importance of Exercise

In consultation with my parents and medical team, we thought it was best to avoid a potential unnecessary surgery, so I had to do physical therapy on my knee. Part of the doctor's orders were I couldn't run or jump for at least 6 months, maybe more if I had any setbacks.

This drove me crazy because I love to run and jump. I missed several great summer camps and couldn't play in any basketball leagues. This was a very sad period for me. There was no way for me to train in Taekwondo or for basketball.

THIS WAS HORRIBLE!

My doctor told me under the best-case scenario, I might be ready to play basketball by the time the next high school season starts (my sophomore year), but I still might not be one hundred percent healed.

I had to alter my routine to stay in shape because I couldn't run. As part of my physical therapy, I did lots of leg exercises. I progressed to more difficult exercises as my knee improved. To get cardio training in, I could walk and ride a stationary bike. I could also do sit ups and light upper body weightlifting, but I had to be careful with my knee.

By the time my sophomore basketball season started, I wasn't fully healed. In consultation with my medical team, it was decided I could play basketball, but I had to stop if I had any setbacks with my knee. I did aggravate my knee some, but my doctor felt it was good enough for me to participate the full season. My parents watched me closely the entire time.

MY RESILIENT WIN

After basketball season ended, I continued with physical therapy for a few months and my knee fully healed. The fact that I was limited in how much exercise I could do for an extended period of time made me appreciate the ability to exercise much more. I was very happy when I finally had zero knee pain.

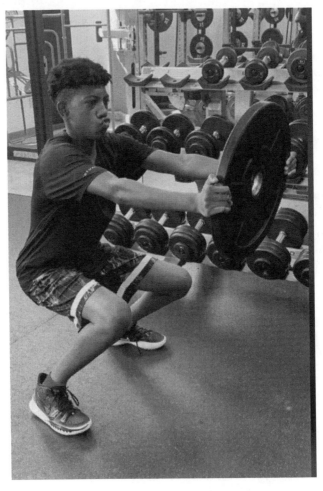

Exercising makes me strong

The Importance of Exercise

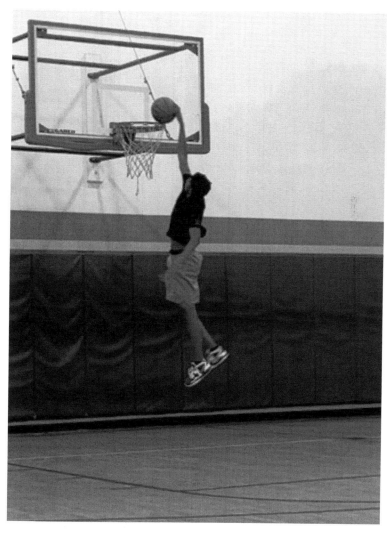

Dunking a basketball

Chapter 13
My Special Hydration Formula: Bradleyaid

It's extra important for anyone who has symptoms of inflammatory bowel disease to stay well hydrated. Whether I'm about to exercise, in the middle of a workout, or I'm done exercising, I keep myself well hydrated with water. However, sometimes I want something more than water. Many athletes drink sugary sports drinks to refuel during workouts or refresh themselves after working out. But I can't have processed sugar, and I'm allergic to soy, gluten, and dairy. As for diet sports drinks, most are loaded with things my body can't have (even if there's no added sugar). But I've solved this issue!

Hydration is important

My mom found a specific carbohydrate electrolyte drink recipe, and I find it works in keeping me well hydrated.

"SCD Electrolyte drink:

- 1 quart boiled water
- 2 tbsp. honey
- 1/4 tsp. of salt
- 1/4 tsp. baking soda

Can be kept in refrigerator for 24 hours and then a new batch should be made."[1]

Because I wanted more flavor and less salt, I altered the recipe above from Elaine Gottschall's work,[2] and created "Bradleyaid." I usually bring it to my practices, games, and athletic camps. It refreshes me.

---

[1] "SCD Electrolyte Drink," Kirkton Press Inc., accessed March 26, 2024, https://breakingtheviciouscycle.info/scd-electrolyte-drink

[2] Elaine Gottschall B.A., M.Sc., *Breaking the Vicious Cycle, Intestinal Health Through Diet*, (Baltimore, Ontario, Canada: Kirkton Press, Fifteenth Printing, December 2014).

Bradleyaid

Ingredients:

1. 2 organic oranges
2. 1/8th of a teaspoon of baking soda
3. 1/8th of a teaspoon of kosher sea salt
4. Two teaspoons of honey, but sometimes I use more
5. 20 ounces of water (spring or purified water)

How to make Bradleyaid

1. Squeeze the juice out of two oranges into a measuring cup.
2. Remove any seeds and pulp with a strainer by pouring the contents from the measuring cup, through a strainer and into a large cup or sports bottle. Discard the seeds and pulp.
3. Add 1/8th of a teaspoon of baking soda to the large cup or sports bottle.
4. Add 1/8th of a teaspoon of kosher sea salt to the large cup or sports bottle.
5. Add two teaspoons of honey to the large cup or sports bottle.

MY RESILIENT WIN

6. Add 20 ounces of spring or purified water into the large cup or sports bottle.
7. Stir the contents of the large cup or vigorously shake the contents of the sports bottle (with the lid closed) until the contents are thoroughly mixed.
8. Refrigerate or serve.

Since this has no preservatives in it, I don't let it sit out at room temperature for more than a few hours and make sure I use all of the Bradleyaid stored in a refrigerator within 24 hours.

Chapter 14
Alternative Treatments

I have to state again not everyone responds well to common treatments for inflammatory bowel disease (IBD), and not everyone can follow the specific carbohydrate diet. This is part of why IBD is so difficult. But newer methods to potentially treat IBD like stem cell therapy and hyperbaric oxygen therapy (HBOT) are being studied as science advances.

Stem Cell Therapy

Stem cells are used to treat IBD by helping repair the colon and reduce inflammation. Some evidence shows patients with IBD experienced a reduction of their symptoms or even remission. But this is still experimental.

In one study on stem cell therapy for Crohn's disease, "only a fraction of patients achieve and remain in remission for a long duration."[1]

Hyperbaric Oxygen Therapy (HBOT)

Hyperbaric oxygen therapy involves breathing pure oxygen in a special pressurized chamber. This increases oxygen levels in the blood and tissues, helping reduce inflammation and speed up healing. While some patients reported benefits, HBOT is still considered experimental for IBD. "To realize a simple treatment like hyperbaric oxygen therapy could have life-changing benefits for these patients is very exciting."[2]

Though these treatments show promise, they aren't widely available yet, and doctors need to study them more to understand how they work best. Stem cell therapy and HBOT offer hope for better managing ulcerative colitis and Crohn's disease in the future. Hopefully, scientific research proves a medical breakthrough for inflammatory bowel disease.

---

[1] Liam Connolly, "UC Davis Health leads study on promising stem cell-based therapy for Crohn's disease," January 29, 2024, https://health.ucdavis.edu/news/headlines/uc-davis-health-leads-study-on-promising-stem-cell-based-therapy-for-crohns-disease/2024/01

[2] "How Does Hyperbaric Oxygen Therapy Help Treat IBD?" April 2023, Northwestern Medicine, https://www.nm.org/healthbeat/medical-advances/how-does-hyperbaric-oxygen-therapy-help-treat-IBD

Chapter 15
I Defeated Ulcerative Colitis

After sticking to the specific carbohydrate diet, within several months, my IBD symptoms were gone. But I had to deal with several flare-ups over my first few years on the diet. In the years since my last flare up, I've not taken any prescription medication for ulcerative colitis. I've eliminated my IBD symptoms with diet and a daily over the counter probiotic (VSL3).

In the years since I've been on the specific carbohydrate diet, my health has been great. At times, I've tested myself by having some foods that are not compliant with the diet. I've been able to do this without experiencing any symptoms of inflammatory bowel disease.

One such test I've done multiple times is having French fried potatoes from Five Guys burgers. My mom didn't let me eat a lot, but on a few occasions, my dad let me have as much as I wanted, and I didn't get sick.

MY RESILIENT WIN

My mom researched Five Guys and since their French fries are cooked in 100% peanut oil, she felt we could test them out. Had their fries been made using corn or soy oil like some restaurants, I wouldn't have tried them. I avoid canola oil as it has been shown to increase inflammation in the body in some studies. I'm not supposed to eat potatoes on the specific carbohydrate diet, but combining potatoes with corn, soy or canola oil would be multiple negative factors and more likely to make me sick.

Since I didn't get sick from eating French fries from Five Guys burger restaurant, periodically to this day, I eat them with no problems. Also, periodically, like twice a month maximum, my parents make French fried potatoes for me by either frying them on a stove top or crisping them in an air fryer. I've been able to enjoy potato French fries each time without getting sick. Sometimes, to make French fries less starchy, we soak cut fries in water overnight. But often, we'll just cut the potatoes, cook them immediately, then I'll eat them.

To be careful and avoid the potential of any IBD flare ups, I don't eat foods forbidden by the specific carbohydrate diet very often, but it's reassuring to know I can have some of the foods I love at times and potentially not get sick. If I eat bad foods, moderation is key.

My teeth

The specific carbohydrate diet has changed my life. It's not just good for getting rid of my IBD symptoms, but I got several unexpected benefits. One big win has been my dental health. Ever since I stopped eating processed sugar, I haven't had a single cavity. It's crazy how what you eat can have such a big impact on your health.

Teens Managing the Specific Carbohydrate Diet

Following any healthy diet might be hard for teens and pre-teens, because it's also hard for adults. Face it, people like to eat foods that taste good. People also want convenience. My dad ate a whole large pizza once and was mad he was two pounds heavier the next day. I don't know why he even bothered to weigh himself.

Sticking to a healthy diet is challenging since food is a common focal point of social gathering, school functions and sporting events. But I've figured out how to have fun without eating bad food. I've become good at picking healthy foods for me when I go out to eat with friends.

I can enjoy meals without sacrificing my health, whether I'm at home or at a restaurant. I do this by choosing recipes that use wholesome, unprocessed ingredients, and don't have anything I'm allergic to in them. If the food fully complies with the specific carbohydrate diet, that's an added benefit. As I've discovered, a lot of restaurants are good at handling specific requests because of dietary restrictions.

I like experimenting with healthy dishes I know won't make me sick and learning about new tastes and ways to cook. In addition to supporting my body with good nutrition, I've broadened my tastes to include homemade yogurt and fermented vegetables like sauerkraut.

I also have grain-free baked goods and stews. I am creative with my meals, and they bring me enjoyment. There's a lot of diversity present in the specific carbohydrate diet.

The specific carbohydrate diet has had a large impact on me. I've restored control of my health and got relief from the symptoms of inflammatory bowel disease by using this eating strategy. I've found that, despite eating non-compliant foods at times, my gut is stronger than I thought. It's great I can eat non-compliant foods at times in moderation without worrying about having flare-ups.

Advantages of the specific carbohydrate diet

The advantages of the specific carbohydrate diet go beyond treating symptoms. They also include better dental health, increased scholastic aptitude and general wellbeing. The SCD has given me a feeling of control over my own health as a teenager facing the challenges of adolescence and managing a chronic health condition. I've welcomed the path towards quality health through good decision-making, smart meal planning and preparation, and a network of family, friends and medical experts who are always there to help me.

Support is needed

My parents, grandparents, friends and doctors really supported me, or I don't know how I would have handled ulcerative colitis. I'm so grateful for getting the emotional support I needed. I've got it good! My resilience paid off.

My reward for resilience is good health!

My parents gave me some extra rewards because they know I love basketball and was traumatized when I physically couldn't make it through a basketball camp. They also know I love the Miami Heat and Dwyane Wade is my favorite basketball player. So, when I was physically healthy, my parents arranged that I'd attend Celebrity Sports Academy's Dwyane Wade Basketball Camp. I also got to attend a luncheon with Mr. Wade and got a nice picture with him. A year later, I got to play Mr. Wade 1 on 1 in basketball (and lost 2-0). A few years later I got to play NBA All-Star Jimmy Butler of the Miami Heat 1 on 1 and lost 2-1 (because Mr. Butler let me score once). Thanks mom and dad, these are memories of a lifetime!

BE RESILIENT!

MY RESILIENT WIN

BE RESILIENT!

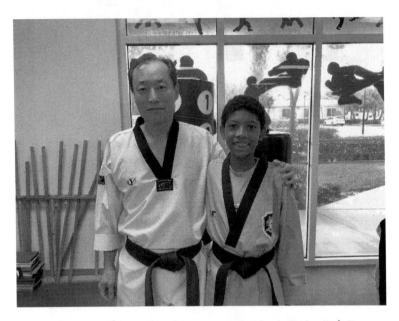

I earned my 2nd Degree International Black Belt (2nd Degree Dan) 15 months after being diagnosed with ulcerative colitis. I'm pictured here with Master Han of U.S. Pro Taekwondo at his Taekwondo training center in Jupiter, Florida in June of 2018. Master Han is a former Korean National and Military Taekwondo champion and has trained many of the world's best martial artists.

BE RESILIENT!

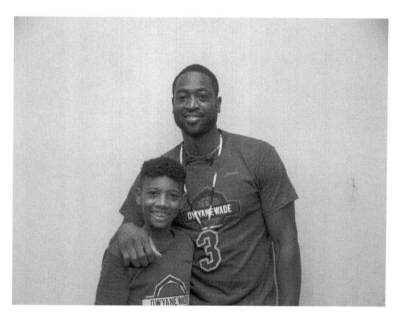

When I was 11 years old, I got to meet NBA Hall of Fame player, Dwyane Wade. It was the first basketball camp I could make it through physically after being diagnosed with ulcerative colitis, and one month after I earned my 2nd Degree International Black Belt in Taekwondo.

MY RESILIENT WIN

BE RESILIENT!

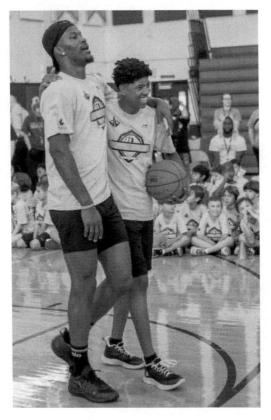

Pictured with NBA All-Star Jimmy Butler of the Miami Heat at Celebrity Sports Academy's Jimmy Butler Basketball Camp in August of 2023. Mr. Butler posted a cover photo of me and him on his official Instagram page.[1]

---

[1] "Jimmy Butler," Instagram, August 28, 2023, https://www.instagram.com/reel/Cwf76x4IFwJ/?igsh=MXZ1N2FvY3h6YmFvYg%3D%3D

I Defeated Ulcerative Colitis

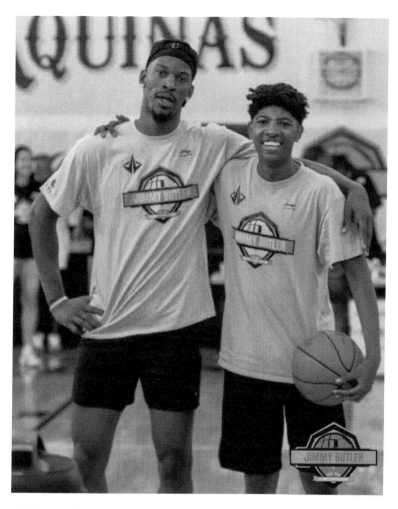

Videos of me playing against Mr. Butler went viral online in posts by The Bleacher Report[1] and NBA Central.[2]

---

[1] "The Bleacher Report," Instagram, August 28, 2023, https://www.instagram.com/p/CwgVYwrJho6/?igsh=am14eTI4OHo3ZTAw&img_index=2
[2] "NBA Central," X, August 28, 2023, https://x.com/TheDunkCentral/status/1696250777012990308

My Resilient Win
A Poem

Resilient through the trauma
resilience and time
if I am resilient
all will be fine

Resilient through the fire
the lightning and the rain
resilience through the silence
you're gonna feel the pain

Resilient keep on fighting
the agony gets worse
the suffering is lonely
I'm bleeding and it hurts

Resilience it's a battle
It's hard to sleep at night
I've got a heavy burden
few understand my plight

Resilient keep the stride
'cause God is on my side
resilient I am bruised
but God won't let me lose

Resilient how I cry
the salt is in my eyes
the crust is on my face
I must pick up the pace

Resilience for the win
resilience at just ten
a monumental hurdle
but my resilient win

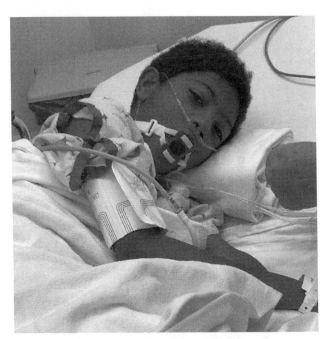

BE RESILIENT!

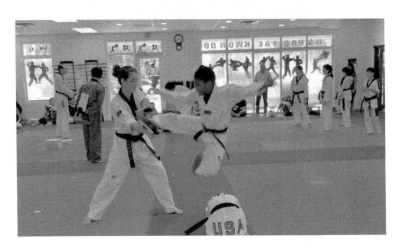

The End

My Resilient Win

Continue for a Preview of My Next Book

A Preview of My Next Book

Saving the World through Financial Literacy and Behavioral Finance

Bradley Collier

A lack of financial literacy is one of the biggest failures in the world! It's time to fix this – the time is now!

--Bradley Collier

A Preview:
How I'll Help Save The World

Beyond the nine-inch scar on his stomach from his sixth emergency surgery, my dad has experienced a great deal of pain. The real scars are the ones you can't see, the ones in his mind. He really understands our family's history, and it haunts him. He says the pain is far worse than any of the surgeries he's had.

Daddy's mother died broke, his father died broke, and his brother died broke. They needed help from friends and family just to avoid being homeless at the end of their lives. It was undignified at best and humiliating at worst. My dad swore that wouldn't be our fate. He's all about planning and working hard so we can live comfortably, and not worry about money.

Financial literacy and behavioral finance are keys to growing wealth and preserving it

While daddy is proud of his and mommy's success, my success, and that of our ancestors, success is not enough. Though success is not necessarily measured in money, you need money to live, and money can help you thrive. I don't think everyone has to aim to be super-rich, but to live comfortably, you need cash.

You see, I have a long history of ancestors who were successful in many ways and made a good amount of money. Many failed to save and invest for the future. And most wasted lots of money to impress others and feed their ego.

When marriages ended, kids got cut off from the possibility of inheriting anything because the dad's only focus became his new family. This made it more difficult for some kids, and it helped destroy others.

Many in my family were addicted to spending money, like it gave them a surge of dopamine, the "feel good" hormone. Feeling the need to fill a psychological

A Preview: How I'll Help Save The World

void by needless spending, possibly fuels many bad purchases. This is like, literally, starting money on fire. Then, when they got sick, disaster struck.

Daddy has done better financially than many because he's planned for the long term. He made me promise to do the same. I must live below my means and save and invest for the future. Yes, I can have nice things, but they must be within reason. And I must give back to society and help others achieve prosperity. I won't repeat my family's mistakes. Instead, I'll learn from them and grow.

I've been called to help lead a revolution. Part of my calling is to help educate people on financial literacy and behavioral finance. This is how I will help save the world.

-Bradley Collier

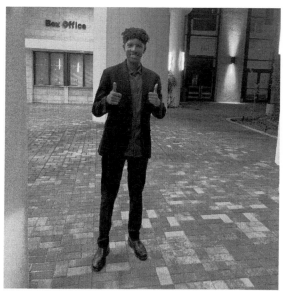

References

1. Olivia Casey and Frederick W. Miller, "Autoimmunity Has Reached Epidemic Levels. We Need Urgent Action to Address it." Scientific American, A Division of Springer Nature America, Inc., December 1, 2023.
https://www.scientificamerican.com/article/autoimmunity-has-reached-epidemic-levels-we-need-urgent-action-to-address-it/
2. Inflammatory Bowel Disease," Yale Medicine, accessed online July 26, 2024,
https://www.yalemedicine.org/conditions/inflammatory-bowel-disease
3. Mayo Clinic Staff, "Inflammatory bowel disease (IBD)," Mayo Clinic, September 3, 2022, https://www.mayoclinic.org/diseases-conditions/inflammatory-bowel-disease/symptoms-causes/syc-20353315
4. "2024 Best U.S. High Schools," U.S. News & World Report, accessed online April 10, 2024,
https://www.usnews.com/education/best-high-schools/florida/districts/the-school-district-of-palm-beach-county/suncoast-community-high-school-5380
5. "Can modern lifestyle affect chances of inflammatory bowel disease?" Medical News Today, Last medically reviewed on March 13, 2024.
https://www.medicalnewstoday.com/articles/320283
6. "Gastroenterology," The Free Dictionary by Farlex, accessed online February 7, 2024
https://www.thefreedictionary.com/gastroenterology
7. "Phlebotomy Technician," Mayo Clinic College of Medicine and Science, Mayo Foundation for Medical Education and Research., accessed online March 9, 2024,
https://college.mayo.edu/academics/explore-health-care-careers/careers-a-z/phlebotomy-technician/

References

8. "Ulcerative Colitis," The Johns Hopkins University, The Johns Hopkins Hospital, and Johns Hopkins Health System, accessed online June 3, 2024, https://www.hopkinsmedicine.org/health/conditions-and-diseases/ulcerative-colitis
9. "Ulcerative Colitis vs Crohn's Disease," UCLA Health, accessed online June 3, 2024, https://www.uclahealth.org/medical-services/gastro/ibd/patient-resources/ulcerative-colitis-vs-crohns-disease
10. "Ulcerative Colitis," The Johns Hopkins University, The Johns Hopkins Hospital, and Johns Hopkins Health System, accessed June 3, 2024, https://www.hopkinsmedicine.org/health/conditions-and-diseases/ulcerative-colitis
11. "Ulcerative Colitis," Michael M. Phillips, MD, David Zieve, MD, MHA, Brenda Conway, Editorial Director, and the A.D.A.M., Editorial team, Penn Medicine, Philadelphia, PA, Last Reviewed on 2/6/2022, accessed online April 9, 2024, https://www.pennmedicine.org/for-patients-and-visitors/patient-information/conditions-treated-a-to-z/ulcerative-colitis
12. Stephanie Watson, medically reviewed by Mikhail Yakubov, MD, "Ulcerative Colitis and Dehydration," Healthline Media, April 16, 2021, https://www.healthline.com/health/ulcerative-colitis/ulcerative-colitis-and-dehydration-what-to-know
13. Stephanie Watson, medically reviewed by Avi Varma, MD, MPH, AAVHIVS, FAAFP, "Everything to Know About Autoimmune Diseases," Healthline, March 4, 2024, https://www.healthline.com/health/autoimmune-disorders
14. Hedy Marks, Medically Reviewed by Poonam Sachdev, MD, "What Is Holistic Medicine and How Does It Work?", WebMD, November 16, 2023, https://www.webmd.com/balance/what-is-holistic-medicine
15. "Blood Tests," FARE (Food Allergy Research & Education), accessed online April 10, 2024, https://www.foodallergy.org/resources/blood-tests
16. "The Specific Carbohydrate Diet," Stanford Medicine, accessed online February 5, 2024. https://med.stanford.edu/content/dam/sm/gastroenterology/documents/IBD/CarbDiet%20PDF%20final.pdf

17. "Specific Carbohydrate Diet (SCD)" Cleveland Clinic, Last reviewed by a Cleveland Clinic medical professional on 07/19/2022, Copyright© 2024. accessed February 5, 2024. https://my.clevelandclinic.org/health/treatments/23543-scd-specific-carbohydrate-diet
18. Elaine Gottschall B.A., M.Sc., Breaking the Vicious Cycle, Intestinal Health Through Diet, (Baltimore, Ontario, Canada: Kirkton Press, Fifteenth Printing, December 2014).
19. Mary Jane Brown, PhD, RD, medically reviewed by Adam Bernstein, MD, ScD, "Does Sugar Cause Inflammation in the Body?," Healthline, updated on February 26, 2024, accessed online April 10, 2024, https://www.healthline.com/nutrition/sugar-and-inflammation
20. Eve M. Glazier, MD, and Elizabeth Ko, MD, "Initial Studies link added sugar and IBD," UCLA Health, February 26, 2021, https://www.uclahealth.org/news/initial-studies-link-added-sugar-and-ibd
21. Ulcerative colitis flare-ups: 5 tips to manage them, July 19, 2023. The Mayo Clinic. https://www.mayoclinic.org/diseases-conditions/ulcerative-colitis/in-depth/ulcerative-colitis-flare-up/art-20120410
22. Camille Peri, Medically Reviewed by Neha Pathak, MD, FACP, DipABLM on May 3, 2024, "6 Benefits of Exercise for Ulcerative Colitis," https://www.webmd.com/ibd-crohns-disease/ulcerative-colitis/uc-exercise
23. Kathryn Whitbourne, Medically Reviewed by Tyler Wheeler, MD on August 12, 2022, "Ulcerative Colitis and Join Pain," WebMD, https://www.webmd.com/ibd-crohns-disease/ulcerative-colitis/ulcerative-colitis-joint-pain
24. "SCD Electrolyte Drink," Kirkton Press Inc., accessed March 26, 2024, https://breakingtheviciouscycle.info/scd-electrolyte-drink
25. Elaine Gottschall B.A., M.Sc., Breaking the Vicious Cycle, Intestinal Health Through Diet, (Baltimore, Ontario, Canada: Kirkton Press, Fifteenth Printing, December 2014).

References

26. Liam Connolly, "UC Davis Health leads study on promising stem cell-based therapy for Crohn's disease," January 29, 2024, https://health.ucdavis.edu/news/headlines/uc-davis-health-leads-study-on-promising-stem-cell-based-therapy-for-crohns-disease/2024/01
27. "How Does Hyperbaric Oxygen Therapy Help Treat IBD?" April 2023, Northwestern Medicine, https://www.nm.org/healthbeat/medical-advances/how-does-hyperbaric-oxygen-therapy-help-treat-IBD
28. "Jimmy Butler," Instagram, August 28, 2023, https://www.instagram.com/reel/Cwf76x4IFwJ/?igsh=MXZ1N2FvY3h6YmFvYg%3D%3D
29. "The Bleacher Report," Instagram, August 28, 2023, https://www.instagram.com/p/CwgVYwrJho6/?igsh=am14eTI4OHo3ZTAw&img_index=2
30. "NBA Central," X, August 28, 2023, https://x.com/TheDunkCentral/status/1696250777012990308

About the Author

Bradley Collier was born in New York City and lives in West Palm Beach, Florida. He is an author, student, and athlete. He hopes to make the world a better place.

He is an AP Scholar with Distinction and was honored by The College Board's National African American Scholar Recognition Program. He is a member of the National Honor Society and served as teen legislative chair for the Palm Beach Chapter of Jack and Jill of America, Inc. He is a 2nd Degree International Black Belt in Taekwondo, and a basketball and track athlete.

Bradley was selected by the AP Government Department Head of Suncoast Community High School in Riviera Beach, Florida, to present his project titled, "*A Student Athlete's Guide To Successfully Manage Their Time*," to students of Bethune Elementary School, JFK Middle School, and parents. He is a member of Future Business Leaders of America, The Black Student Union, Economic Leaders of America, and Technology Student Association.

Bradley collected and donated a large amount of Lego toys to Roots Strong, LLC. The toys were sent to children in Africa, The Caribbean, and urban areas in the U.S. He is a Certified Unity User Artist, mastering Unity Technologies engine after completing over 150 hours of training and software use.

Bradley earned certificates from the University of Michigan in Finance for Everyone, Smart Tools for Decision-Making and Coursera in Deep Learning AI, AI for Everyone. Bradley is dedicated to getting good grades and plans to attend college after high school. His goals are to promote financial literacy and good health.

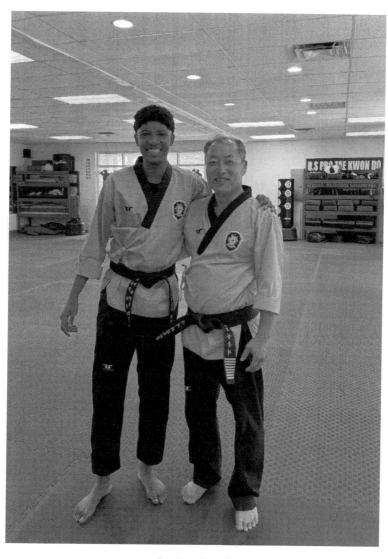
Be Resilient!

Made in the USA
Middletown, DE
27 July 2024